Cutaneous Disorders of Pregnancy

Kelly H. Tyler
Editor

Cutaneous Disorders of Pregnancy

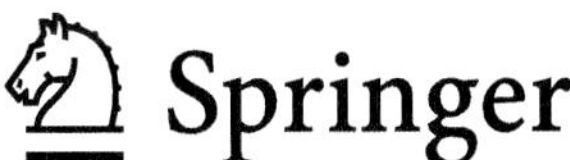

Editor
Kelly H. Tyler, MD
Internal Medicine, Division of Dermatology
Ohio State University
Columbus, OH
USA

ISBN 978-3-030-49287-8 ISBN 978-3-030-49285-4 (eBook)
https://doi.org/10.1007/978-3-030-49285-4

This Springer imprint is published by the registered company Springer Nature Switzerland AG
The registered company address is: Gewerbestrasse 11, 6330 Cham, Switzerland

To my funny and flexible husband Jaret for putting up with me through two residencies and a surprise career change. Also, to my son Dean who always makes me laugh. I hope you never lose your zest for life!

Preface

I started my medical career as a general obstetrician/gynecologist. At the University of Alabama at Birmingham, I trained under major textbook authors and some of the most renowned Maternal Fetal Medicine physicians in the field. Coming out of training, I felt very comfortable with medication safety in pregnancy and prescribing for pregnant patients. As an obstetrician, you get accustomed to the fact that most of what you do is based on expert opinion, and most medications do not have robust pregnancy data. Researchers can't do studies on pregnant patients, so data on medication safety are derived from such sources as case reports of incidental exposures and pregnancy registries. For physicians in other fields who spend the majority of their training looking at high-quality data, this can be disconcerting, and it makes prescribing during pregnancy even more difficult.

When I got out into private practice, skin disease in pregnancy was more challenging for me than medication safety. Much of an Ob/Gyn resident's time is spent in training for surgeries and deliveries, and topics such as skin disease and dermatoses of pregnancy were a small fraction of my education. In order to properly treat my patients, I decided to come up with a plan to address this deficit in my knowledge. I approached Dr. Matthew Zirwas, the residency director at the Ohio State University dermatology residency program at the time, with the intention of scheduling some time to shadow in clinic and learn more about skin disease in pregnancy, vulvar disease, and common dermatologic conditions. He rightfully advised me that a thorough understanding of dermatology would require more than shadowing, and much to my surprise, he suggested I apply for a residency. At the time, I had already been out in practice for 5 years, so going back to training seemed daunting, not to mention that dermatology is considered one of the most competitive residencies.

With nothing to lose, I poured my extra time, evenings, and vacation days into shadowing in the dermatology resident clinic, volunteering at the local free clinic for dermatology, and writing review articles that addressed the overlap between dermatology and obstetrics/gynecology. Perhaps the most challenging part of the process was trying to get an Electronic Residency Application Service (ERAS) token from the Graduate Medical Education office at my alma mater, Tulane University Medical Center. As you can imagine, not many past graduates call almost

10 years later stating they will be applying for another residency, so they were a bit confused at first. To make a long story short, I was fortunate enough to match into the dermatology residency program at the Ohio State, and this book is part of fulfilling my mission of increasing education about skin disease in the female patient. It was a long, interesting, and rewarding journey, and I want others to benefit from my experience.

My hope is for this book to provide guidance for anyone caring for a pregnant patient who has normal but concerning skin changes, a pre-existing dermatologic condition, or a pregnancy-specific dermatosis. With the proper knowledge and resources, all healthcare professionals should feel confident providing adequate and safe treatments that can benefit both the mother and the fetus.

Columbus, OH, USA Kelly H. Tyler

Acknowledgments

I would like to acknowledge Dr. Benjamin Kaffenberger and Dr. Steven Helms for generously contributing photos for this book.

I would also like to acknowledge and express my gratitude to all of the authors who spent countless hours compiling data and composing such eloquent chapters.

Contents

Part I Pregnancy-Specific Skin Changes and Disorders

1 **Physiologic Skin Changes in Pregnancy** 3
Mark A. Bechtel

2 **Pregnancy Dermatoses** 13
Sabrina Shearer, Alecia Blaszczak, and Jessica Kaffenberger

Part II Pre-Existing Skin Disease in Pregnancy

3 **Psoriasis** 43
Daisy Danielle Yan and Lisa Pappas-Taffer

4 **Autoimmune Connective Tissue Diseases** 51
Daisy Danielle Yan and Lisa Pappas-Taffer

5 **Atopic Dermatitis in Pregnancy**. 59
Blake Friedman and Lionel Bercovitch

6 **Acne and Rosacea in Pregnancy** 75
Casey A. Spell, Hannah R. Badon, Amy Flischel,
and Robert T. Brodell

Part III Skin Cancer and Dermatologic Surgery During Pregnancy

7 **Skin Cancer in Pregnancy** 89
Jennifer Villasenor-Park

8 **Dermatologic Surgery in Pregnancy** 113
Jennifer Villasenor-Park

Conclusion 123

Index. 125

Contributors

Hannah R. Badon, MD Department of Dermatology, University of Mississippi Medical Center, Jackson, MS, USA

Mark A. Bechtel, MD Department of Internal Medicine, Division of Dermatology, Ohio State University, Columbus, OH, USA

Lionel Bercovitch, MD Department of Dermatology, Warren Alpert Medical School of Brown University, Providence, RI, USA

Division of Pediatric Dermatology, Hasbro Children's Hospital, Providence, RI, USA

Department of Medicine, Women and Infannts Hospital, Providence, RI, USA

Alecia Blaszczak, PhD Division of Dermatology, Ohio State University, Gahanna, OH, USA

Robert T. Brodell, MD Department of Dermatology, University of Mississippi Medical Center, Jackson, MS, USA

Amy Flischel, MD Northwestern Medical Group, Vernon Hills, IL, USA

Blake Friedman, MD Department of Dermatology, Warren Alpert Medical School of Brown University, Providence, RI, USA

Jessica Kaffenberger, MD Division of Dermatology, Ohio State University, Gahanna, OH, USA

Lisa Pappas-Taffer, MD Department of Dermatology, University of Pennsylvania, Philadelphia, PA, USA

Sabrina Shearer, MD Department of Dermatology, Duke University, Durham, NC, USA

Casey A. Spell, BS University of Mississippi Medical School, Jackson, MS, USA

Jennifer Villasenor-Park, MD, PhD Department of Dermatology, University of Pennsylvania, Philadelphia, PA, USA

Daisy Danielle Yan, BA Department of Dermatology, University of Pennsylvania, Philadelphia, PA, USA

Introduction

Treating pregnant patients presents a challenge for all physicians and healthcare professionals, regardless of specialty. Due to concern for side effects on the fetus, many physicians or practitioners tend to err on the side of caution, often resulting in undertreatment. Skin disorders in pregnancy can be particularly challenging, not only because physiologic skin changes in pregnancy that seem abnormal may actually represent normal variants, but also because dermatology is not always a specialty that gets adequate attention during routine medical education. Perhaps one of the more challenging aspects of treating skin disease during pregnancy is that most data on medication safety in pregnancy are based on incidental exposures, case reports, and expert opinion, so there are no controlled human studies, and we must rely on animal data in many cases.

Classification of medication safety in pregnancy and lactation has evolved over the years, and it underwent a major change in 2015. Historically, we used the Federal Drug Administration (FDA) pregnancy categories (Table 1.1) as a main source of information about medication safety in pregnancy. Each medication was assigned a letter, indicating its level of safety for use in pregnancy. Sixty six percent of drugs were FDA Pregnancy Category C [1], which is described as: Risk cannot be ruled out; human studies may or may not show risk; potential benefits may justify potential risk. That non-specific description, which applied to the majority of medications, is not reassuring, and most practitioners who did not routinely treat pregnant patients felt uncomfortable prescribing a category C medication.

This classification system was imprecise because the potential risk of the drug is not a global risk and often depends on which trimester the exposure happened. The stages of prenatal development are as follows: pre-implantation – 0–2 weeks, embryonic/organogenesis – 2–8 weeks, and fetal – 9th week to birth. Avoiding teratogenic medications during the embryonic period is the most important, but the brain, teeth, and bones do remain susceptible after 9 weeks. When prescribing for women of childbearing age, it is critical to remember that a home pregnancy test may not be positive until up to 5 weeks after conception, so any woman who is not on contraception and could potentially become pregnant should be treated with medications that are safe to use during pregnancy.

For most dermatologic conditions, topical medications are the safest choice and should be considered first-line. Studies of various topicals estimate systemic absorption to range from less than 4–25% [2]. For topical medications, using them on a smaller body surface area, using the option with the lowest potency, and avoiding occlusion will decrease systemic absorption. Systemic medications can be used when necessary if the practitioner is knowledgeable about safety ratings and high-risk periods during pregnancy. Common systemic dermatologic medications that are teratogenic (previous FDA pregnancy category X) and absolutely contraindicated in pregnant patients or those who could become pregnant are isotretinoin, acitretin, and methotrexate.

The new FDA medication safety labeling, which took effect on 6/30/2015 for newly approved medications, includes a fetal risk summary, clinical considerations, and data. Manufacturers of older medications were required to revise labeling and remove letter categories within 3 years of that date [3]. Although the new system gives more specific information, reading and interpreting each summary does require extra work on the part of the treating physician or practitioner. Because many readers will have more experience with the classic FDA pregnancy medication categories, most authors have included those ratings in the sections of each chapter dedicated to treatment.

With proper knowledge of medication safety during pregnancy, physiologic skin changes in pregnancy, pregnancy-specific dermatoses, and common pre-existing skin disorders not specific to pregnancy, any healthcare professional can confidently treat dermatologic conditions in their pregnant patients and avoid unnecessary risks to the mother and fetus that could result from either inappropriate treatment or undertreatment. In the chapters that follow, the authors give a thorough review of the above topics, provide specific information about medication safety for each condition, and present guidelines for safely using dermatologic surgery during pregnancy.

References

1. Sannerstedt R, Lundborg P, Danielsson BR, et al. Drugs during pregnancy: an issue of risk classification and information to prescribers. Drug Saf. 1996;14:69–7.
2. Tyler K, Zirwas M. Pregnancy and dermatologic therapy. J Am Acad Dermatol 2013;68(4):663–1.
3. http://www.fda.gov/drugs/developmentapprovalprocess/developmentresources/labeling/ucm093307.htm.

Part I
Pregnancy-Specific Skin Changes and Disorders

Chapter 1
Physiologic Skin Changes in Pregnancy

Mark A. Bechtel

Introduction

Pregnancy is associated with a variety of physiologic changes that can have a direct impact on the skin. Metabolic, immunologic, and hormonal alterations during pregnancy can impact the appearance and morphology of the skin. These alterations can affect skin pigmentation, cutaneous vasculature, existing cutaneous lesions, hair, and nails. Although some changes can be concerning to the patient and health care providers, most are benign and resolve or improve after delivery. A comprehensive review of the physiologic changes of the skin during pregnancy is provided in this chapter.

Pigmentary Changes

One of the most striking physiologic changes of the skin during pregnancy is the impact on pigmentation. Approximately 90% of pregnant women manifest some form of hyperpigmentation [1, 2]. Hyperpigmentation becomes more prominent during the second half of pregnancy and is often in specific areas and patterns [1, 2].

The linea alba darkens to become the linea nigra, which extends from the xiphoid process to the pubic symphysis [1, 3, 4] (Fig. 1.1). The linea nigra often fades or resolves following delivery, and the cause is unknown. An accentuated darkening of normally hyperpigmented regions of skin can occur during pregnancy as well. This is most apparent in the axillae, genitalia, perineum, and inner thighs [1, 3]. Sometimes darkening of the skin around the areola produces what is termed a

M. A. Bechtel (✉)
Department of Internal Medicine, Division of Dermatology, Ohio State University, Columbus, OH, USA

K. H. Tyler (ed.), *Cutaneous Disorders of Pregnancy*,
https://doi.org/10.1007/978-3-030-49285-4_1

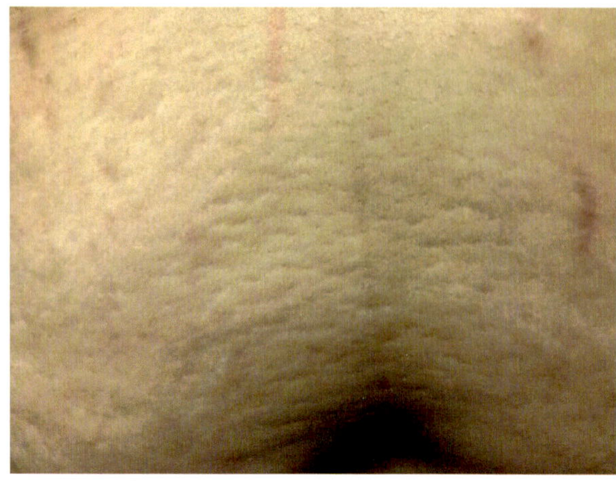

Fig. 1.1 Linea nigra. Linear hyperpigmentation extending to the xiphoid process, which fades postpartum

secondary areola [2, 4]. Darkening of freckles and nevi has been reported during pregnancy, but there may be insufficient evidence to support this observation [5]. Despite the controversy, biopsies should be obtained promptly from any changing nevi during pregnancy that raise concern for malignancy [5].

Pigmentary demarcation lines can develop during pregnancy and present as abrupt transitions from heavily pigmented skin to areas of lighter pigmentation [4]. The demarcation lines are known as Voigt or Futcher lines and present along the posterior legs or upper arms [3]. Resolution after delivery is usually observed, and no treatment is needed [4]. There is no clear etiology for the development of demarcation lines, but an association with peripheral nerves has been suggested [4].

Increased melanogenesis during pregnancy is complex and may be related to increased levels of beta and alpha melanocyte stimulating hormone (MSH), estrogen, and progesterone [3]; however, increased pigmentation may occur early in pregnancy before MSH levels become elevated [1]. Increased pigmentation may also be impacted by increased density of epidermal melanocytes and upregulation of tyrosinase by human placental lipids [1]. Recently, it has been shown that physiologic estrogen (17-beta estradiol) and progesterone reciprocally regulate melanin syntheses. Sex steroid effects on human pigment synthesis are mediated by membrane-bound steroid hormone receptors [6], and estrogen effects are significantly attenuated by the presence of progesterone. This may explain why pregnancy-associated hyperpigmentation primarily occurs in areas with a higher baseline melanocyte density or increased ultraviolet radiation exposure [6].

Melasma (chloasma or mask of pregnancy) is prominent facial hyperpigmentation that develops in up to 70% of pregnant patients [3, 7]. The hyperpigmentation is often symmetric and poorly demarcated. Distribution of melasma may involve the nose and cheeks (malar), the entire central face (centrofacial), or the ramus of the mandible (mandibular) [1, 3, 7] (Fig. 1.2). The depth of melanin deposition varies, which impacts its appearance under a Wood's lamp. The melanin is deposited in the epidermis in 70%, dermal melanophages in 10–15%, and both in 20% [7]. Women

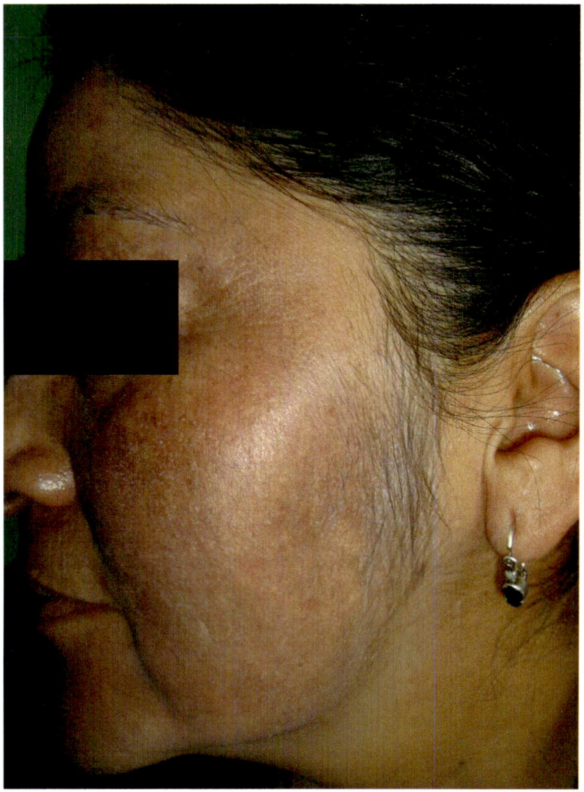

Fig. 1.2 Melasma. Prominent poorly demarcated facial hyperpigmentation of melasma develops in up to 70% of pregnant patients. (Courtesy Benjamin Kaffenberger, MD)

with darker skin are especially affected. Melasma usually improves postpartum, but patients need to be advised that it may recur with subsequent pregnancies or possibly flare with use of estrogen-containing oral contraceptives. Postpartum melasma may persist in 30% of patients despite treatment [7].

High sun protective factor broad spectrum sunscreens with UVA protection may lessen the severity of melasma. Other than sunscreen, most treatments for melasma should be deferred until the postpartum period. Hydroquinone, one of the most common treatments for melasma, has a transcutaneous absorption of 35–45% and distributes rapidly and widely [8]. This raises concern for use during pregnancy and lactation, so it is typically avoided. Tretinoin was a previous Federal Drug Administration (FDA) pregnancy category C (Table 1.1) [9], and studies are conflicting on whether it is teratogenic during the first trimester of pregnancy [9]. The safety data of topical retinoids such as tretinoin and adapalene are limited, and most experts recommend avoiding these during pregnancy [8]. Due to lack of absorption in significant quantities, tretinoin and adapalene are likely safe during lactation [10]. With regard to elective cosmetic laser treatments for melasma, although there are no adverse fetal complications reported, most health care practitioners choose not to perform them during pregnancy [7].

Table 1.1 US Food and Drug Administration pregnancy risk categories

Category	Description
A	Controlled studies show no fetal risk
B	No risk to human fetus despite possible animal risk; or no risk in animal studies and human studies not done
C	Risk cannot be ruled out; human studies have not been performed; animal studies may or may not show risk; potential benefits may justify potential risk
D	Positive evidence of risk to human fetus, but benefits may outweigh risks of drug
X	Contraindicated in pregnancy; there is no reason to risk use of drug in pregnancy

Azelaic acid, another common topical treatment for melasma, is a former FDA pregnancy category B (Table 1.1) drug. In a large double-blind study, azelaic acid 20% had good or excellent results in 65% of patients, similar results to hydroquinone [11]. Azelaic acid is therefore considered a safe, reasonable choice to treat melasma during pregnancy and lactation.

All the above topical treatments are considered safe to treat melasma following pregnancy and lactation. Additional topical treatments to consider for melasma postpartum include triple combination creams (hydroquinone, tretinoin, topical steroid) and kojic acid. Glycolic acid peels, laser, intense pulse light, and topical and oral tranexamic acid are additional therapeutic considerations.

Connective Tissue Changes

Striae gravidarum (stretch marks, striae distensae) develop in up to 90% of Caucasian women and less commonly in Asians and African American women during pregnancy [7]. They appear most often in the second and third trimester and affect the abdomen, breasts, buttocks, thighs, and hips [12]. Initially, striae appear pink or violaceous, but over months they become white, atrophic, and shiny (Fig. 1.3). Risk factors include excessive weight gain during pregnancy, genetic susceptibility, young maternal age, and concomitant use of steroids [7]. Mechanical tension may be important in the pathogenesis, but this is not well defined. Histologically, there is a disruption of dermal connective tissue, including collagen and elastic fibrils [12].

The treatment options for striae gravidarum are suboptimal. Currently, we lack the double-blind randomized clinical trials with large numbers of patients needed to fully evaluate the efficacy and safety of topical therapies and laser devices in preventing and treating striae gravidarum [13]. Topical centella, a plant found in South Asia, along with bitter almond oil massaged into striae may reduce the severity, but evidence is limited. Cocoa butter and olive oil do not demonstrate efficacy [12].

Tretinoin may decrease the severity of erythematous striae by stimulating activity of dermal fibroblasts, but it is pregnancy category C (Table 1.1) and should be deferred until after pregnancy and lactation [12]. Postpartum and after breastfeeding is complete, topical tretinoin cream 0.1% applied nightly for 3 months demonstrated efficacy [14]. Treatment with ablative functional photothermolysis, non-ablative

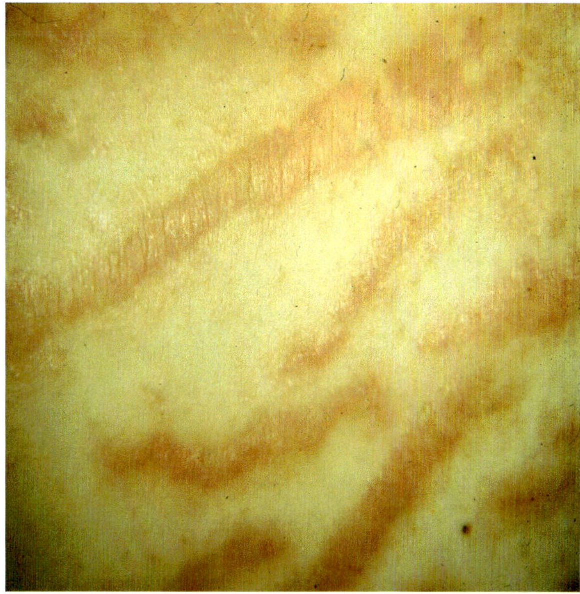

Fig. 1.3 Striae gravidarum. Prominent pink striae gravidarum over the abdomen develop during the second and third trimester

fractional photothermolysis, pulse dye lasers, and intense pulse light have been reported to be beneficial [15]. Recently, the non-ablative fractional laser has demonstrated some efficacy for striae rubra and striae alba [16].

Molluscum fibrosum gravidarum or skin tags are frequent during the second and third trimester [1]. They are 1–5 mm flesh colored papules, which are often pedunculated and occur on the neck, axillae, groin, and inframammary regions [7]. Lesions often regress postpartum and usually do not require treatment during pregnancy. If skin tags persist postpartum and are symptomatic, they can be treated by cryotherapy or snip excision.

Hair and Nail Changes

Postpartum hair shedding, known as telogen effluvium, can result in significant shedding of scalp hair and can be very distressing to the patient (Fig. 1.4). The life span of a hair follicle involves a prolonged growth phase (anagen), involution stage (catagen), and resting phase (telogen). Hair growth is non-synchronized, and approximately 10% of hair follicles are in telogen phase preparing to shed at any given time. During pregnancy, an increased number of hair follicles remain in the anagen phase for longer periods, so there is a significant increase in hair length and hair diameter compared to the non-pregnant patient [17]. After delivery, a rapid transition from anagen to telogen phase occurs. The shedding of hair usually begins 1–5 months after delivery and may continue for up to 1–2 years [3]. Women at risk for androgenetic alopecia (AGA) tend to develop postpartum alopecia, possibly due

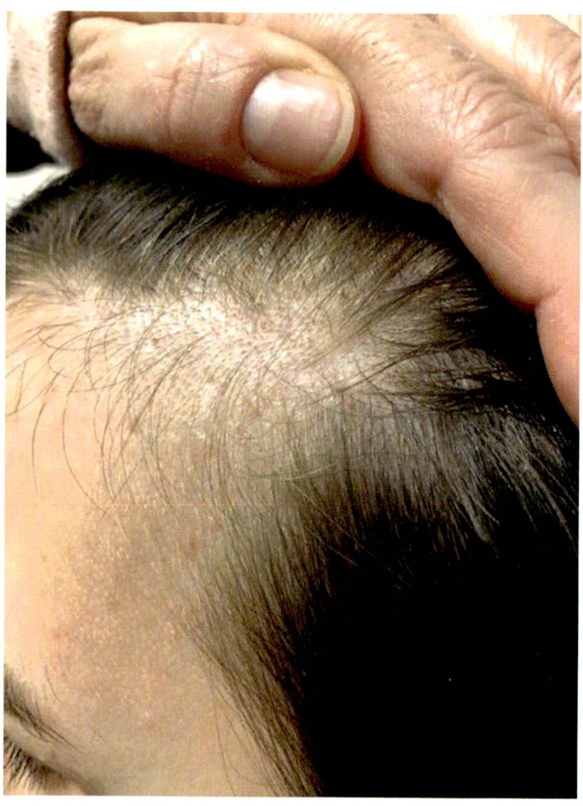

Fig. 1.4 Telogen effluvium. Postpartum shedding of hair from the scalp, telogen effluvium usually begins 1–5 months after delivery

to the shortened anagen phase in AGA. There is no specific treatment for telogen effluvium, but thyroid disease and iron deficiency should be excluded. The prognosis for hair regrowth is excellent, and reassurance is important [3]. It should be noted that hair loss is not impacted by breastfeeding.

Hirsutism, excessive growth of dark, course hair in a male-like pattern, is common during pregnancy and can affect the face, chest, lower abdomen, back, and extremities. It is more apparent in women with darker hair [1, 3]. The onset is in early pregnancy and often regresses within 6 months postpartum [7]. Hirsutism is thought to be secondary to increased placental and ovarian androgens [1]. Severe hirsutism during pregnancy should warrant an endocrine work up for an androgen secreting tumor. If unwanted hair persists beyond 6 months postpartum, laser hair removal can be considered.

Nail growth is increased during pregnancy, and the nails may become brittle and soft. Subungual hyperkeratosis and onycholysis have been noted [18]. Traverse grooves (Beau's lines) and longitudinal melanonychia, linear streaks of darker pigmentation in the nail plate, have been reported [1]. Nail changes may be noted as early as the sixth week of pregnancy [3]. In a large clinical study of nail alterations during pregnancy, leukonychia (white discoloration, 24.4%), onychocryptosis (ingrown nails, 9.0%) and onychoschizia (nail splitting, 9.0%) were the most common [19].

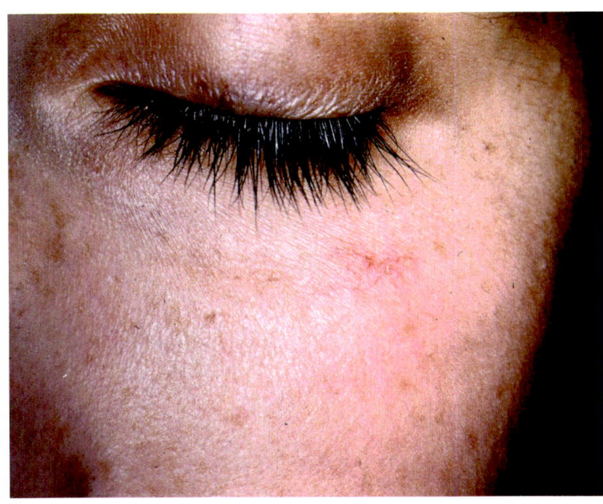

Fig. 1.5 Spider angiomata. Common during pregnancy, spider angiomata manifest as raised telangiectatic puncta with radiating branches

Vascular Changes

Spider angiomata are one of the most common vascular changes of pregnancy. They first appear during the second to fifth months of pregnancy as flat or slightly raised telangiectatic red puncta with surrounding radiating branches [3] (Fig. 1.5). Spider angiomata are noted in areas drained by the superior vena cava (face, neck, arms, and hands) [20]. Approximately two-thirds of Caucasian women may develop spider angiomata during pregnancy, but they are less common in black women [1, 3]. They tend to increase in number and size until delivery and then usually fade by 2 months postpartum [21]. Vascular lesions that persist more than several months after delivery can be treated by fine needle cautery, pulsed dye laser, or intense pulsed light [20].

Palmar erythema is a common vascular change during pregnancy and may be early in onset [3]. Approximately two-thirds of Caucasian patients and one-third of women of color develop palmar erythema [1, 3, 7]. The palmar erythema may present as mottled erythema of the palms or mottling of the thenar or hypothenar eminences and finger pads. Palmar erythema may be associated with a burning sensation [22]. Within 1–2 weeks after delivery, the palmar erythema rapidly resolves [1, 3, 20]. Of note, palmar erythema may also be seen in association with cirrhosis and lupus erythematosus [20].

Granuloma gravidarum or pyogenic granuloma of pregnancy is a benign proliferation of capillaries during pregnancy which often presents on the gingiva [7]. They may present as asymptomatic erythematous fragile papules or nodules on the gingival mucosa, but they may occur on the lip or non- mucosal sites [20] (Fig. 1.6). The most common location is between the teeth or on the buccal or lingual surface [7]. Plaque deposits or gingivitis may be contributing factors [20]. Because the lesions typically undergo spontaneous shrinkage following delivery, they often require only reassurance. Excessive bleeding, tenderness, or irritation may be an indication for treatment. Electrosurgical desiccation, vascular lasers, or excision can

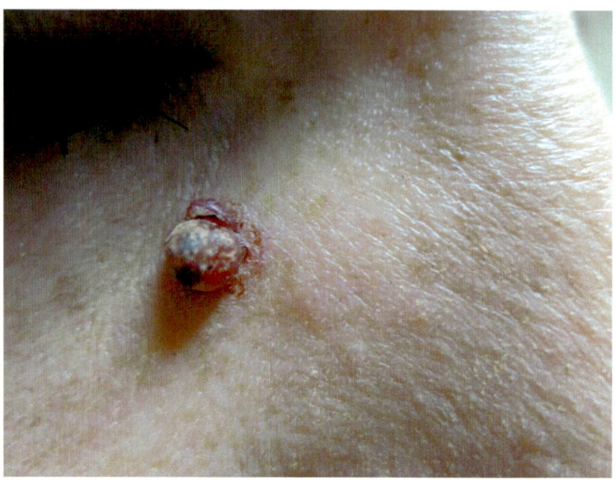

Fig. 1.6 Granuloma gravidarum. Granuloma gravidarum or pyogenic granuloma of pregnancy manifest as friable erythematous vascular papules or nodules

be considered. Post op bleeding is common and can complicate surgical excision [20].

Venous hypertension and venous varicosities during pregnancy are common due to dynamic changes that occur in the maternal cardiovascular system [22]. These include expansion of plasma volume, increased uteroplacental blood flow, increased cardiac output, and decreased peripheral resistance [23]. Hormonal upregulation of substances such as relaxin impacts vascular tone and connective tissue, and estrogen and progesterone activity impact renal water retention [24].

The gravid uterus compresses the femoral and pelvic vessels, resulting in increased venous pressure. Although varicosities during pregnancy are widespread, the saphenous vein is most commonly involved [2]. Varicosities involving the legs, vagina, vulva, and anus occur in approximately 40% of pregnant women and start in the second month [3, 20]. Hemorrhoidal varicosities are common and often symptomatic with pain and thrombosis [3]. Varicosities are most symptomatic during the last trimester and first month postpartum [20]. Aggravating factors include high birthweight of the newborn, constipation, and prolonged straining during delivery [20]. Varicosities of the vestibule and vagina result in a bluish tint of the vaginal mucosa, known as Jacquemier's or Chadwick's sign, which appears around the eighth week of pregnancy [20].

Leg varicosities can be treated with left sided sleeping, leg elevation, compression stockings, and avoidance of prolonged sitting or standing [1–3]. Varicosities of the legs usually improve postpartum, but symptomatic lesions persisting 3 months postpartum can be treated by sclerotherapy or laser [20]. Hemorrhoids can be treated by sitz baths, topical anesthetics, and avoidance of constipation with laxatives [3, 20].

Finally, increased capillary permeability, combined with salt and water retention, results in non-pitting edema of the face and extremities in over half of pregnant patients [1]. Persistent swelling of the hands and face may be a sign of pre-eclampsia [2].

Glandular Activity

Eccrine function is increased during pregnancy and may contribute to dyshidrosis, hyperhidrosis, and miliaria. Apocrine activity may decrease with improvement in Fox-Fordyce disease and potentially hidradenitis suppurativa [7]. Increased eccrine activity is noted at the end of pregnancy but spares the palms [1, 3]. Fox-Fordyce disease and hidradenitis suppurativa may rebound postpartum when apocrine activity increases [3].

Sebaceous gland activity increases late in pregnancy and may exacerbate acne [3]; however, the impact of sebaceous activity on acne is variable with some reports of improvement and worsening [2]. Sebaceous glands on the areola may enlarge starting in the sixth week of pregnancy and are known as Montgomery tubercles [20]. This may be an early sign of pregnancy. Montgomery tubercles are described as brown papules on the areola which represent sebaceous gland hyperplasia and regress postpartum. They provide lubrication for the nipples and areolas for breastfeeding [2]. Montgomery tubercles are noted in 30–50% of pregnant women [3].

Conclusion

Pregnancy is associated with metabolic, hormonal, and immunologic changes that directly impact the skin. These physiologic alterations affect skin pigmentation, connective tissue, the vasculature, hair, and nails. Although sometimes concerning to the patient, the physiologic changes of the skin during pregnancy are usually benign and improve after delivery. It is important for the healthcare provider to be aware of these changes to properly manage appropriate concerns and provide reassurance.

References

1. Geraghty LN, Pomeranz MK. Physiologic changes and dermatoses of pregnancy. Int J Dermatol. 2011;50(7):771–82.
2. Motosko CC, Bieber AK, Pomeranz MK, et al. Physiologic changes in pregnancy: a review of the literature. Int J Womens Dermatol. 2017;3(4):219–24.
3. Tyler KH. Physiologic skin changes during pregnancy. Clin Obstet Gynecol. 2015;58:119–24.
4. Bieber AK, Martires KJ, Stein JA, et al. Pigmentation and pregnancy: knowing what is normal. Obstet Gynecol. 2017;129(1):168–73.
5. Bieber AK, Martires KJ, Driscoll MS, et al. Nevi and pregnancy. J Am Acad Dermatol. 2016;75(4):661–6.
6. Natale CA, Duperret EK, Zhang J, et al. Sex steroids regulate skin pigmentation through nonclassical membrane-bound receptors. Elife. 2016;5:e15104. https://doi.org/10.7554/eLife.15104.

7. Kroumpouzos G. Skin disease in pregnancy and puerperium. In: Gabbe SG, Niebyl JR, Simpson JL, Landon MB, Galan HL, Jauniaux ER, Driscoll DA, editors. Obstetrics: normal and problem pregnancies. 6th ed. Philadelphia: Elsevier/Saunders; 2012. p. 1084–97.
8. Murase JE, Heller MM, Butler DC. Safety of dermatologic medications in pregnancy and lactation: part 1. Pregnancy. J Am Acad Dermatol. 2014;70(3):401.e1–14.
9. Tyler KH. Dermatologic therapy in pregnancy. Clin Obstet Gynecol. 2015;58:112–8.
10. Butler DC, Heller MM, Murase JE. Safety of dermatologic medications in pregnancy and lactation: Part II. Lactation. J Am Acad Dermatol. 2014;70(3):417.e1–10.
11. Balina LM, Graupek K. The treatment of melasma: 20% azelaic acid versus 4% hydroquinone cream. Int J Dermatol. 1991;30:893–5.
12. Korgavkar K, Wang F. Stretch marks during pregnancy: a review of topical prevention. Br J Dermatol. 2014;172(3):606–15. https://doi.org/10.1111/bjd.13426.
13. Al-Himdani S, Vd-Din S, Gilmore S, et al. Striae distensae: a comprehensive review and evidence-based evaluation of prophylaxis and treatment. Br J Dermatol. 2014;170(3):527–47.
14. Rangel O, Aries I, Garcia E, et al. Topical tretinoin 0.1% for pregnancy-related abdominal striae: an open-label, multicenter, prospective study. Adv Ther. 2001;18(4):181–6.
15. Nabatian AS, Khorasani H. Striae. In: Lebwohl MF, Heymann WR, Berth-Jones J, Coulson I, editors. Treatment of skin disease: comprehensive therapeutic strategies. 5th ed. Philadelphia: Elsevier; 2018. p. 794–6.
16. Gokulp H. Long-term results of the treatment of pregnancy-induced striae distensae using a 1550-nm non-ablative fractional laser. J Cosmet Laser Ther. 2017;19(7):378–82.
17. Gizlenti S, Ekmekci JR. The changes in the hair cycle during gestation and the postpartum period. J Eur Acad Dermatol Venereol. 2014;28:878–81.
18. Kar S, Krishnan A, Shivkumar PV. Pregnancy and skin. J Obstet Gynaecol India. 2012;62(3):268–75.
19. Erpolat S, Eser A, Kaygusuz I, et al. Nail alterations during pregnancy: a clinical study. Int J Dermatol. 2016;55:1172–5.
20. Soutou B, Aractingi S. Skin disease in pregnancy. Best Pract Res Clin Obstet Gynaecol. 2015;29(5):732–40.
21. Wong RC, Ellis CN. Physiologic skin changes in pregnancy. J Am Acad Dermatol. 1984;10:929–40.
22. Henry F, Quatresooz P, Valverde-Lopez JC, et al. Blood vessel changes during pregnancy: a review. Am J Clin Dermatol. 2006;7(1):65–9.
23. Osol G, Ko NL, Mandala M. Plasticity of the maternal vasculature during pregnancy. Annu Rev Physiol. 2019;81:89–111.
24. Kepley JM, Mohiuddin SS. Physiology, maternal changes. Treasure Island: StatPearls; 2019; https://www.ncbi.nlm.nih.gov/books/NBK539766/.

Chapter 2
Pregnancy Dermatoses

Sabrina Shearer, Alecia Blaszczak, and Jessica Kaffenberger

Polymorphic Eruption of Pregnancy

Synonyms

(Bourne's) Toxemic rash of pregnancy; Toxic erythema of pregnancy; (Nurse's) Late onset prurigo of pregnancy; *Prurigo of pregnancy; Pruritic urticarial papules and plaques of pregnancy; Erythema multiforme of pregnancy; *Linear IgM dermatosis of pregnancy.

Definition

Polymorphic eruption of pregnancy (PEP) has been recognized in the literature under various names for decades. It was previously known in the United States by the descriptive term "pruritic urticarial papules and plaques of pregnancy" [1]; however, given its myriad of presentations, Holmes et al. coined the nomenclature "polymorphic eruption of pregnancy" in 1982 [2].

---

* Some classifications group these entities with polymorphic eruption of pregnancy (PEP) or as separate dermatoses.

S. Shearer
Department of Dermatology, Duke University, Durham, NC, USA
e-mail: Sabrina.shearer@duke.edu

A. Blaszczak · J. Kaffenberger (✉)
Division of Dermatology, Ohio State University, Gahanna, OH, USA
e-mail: Alecia.blaszczak@osumc.edu; Jessica.kaffenberger@osumc.edu

K. H. Tyler (ed.), *Cutaneous Disorders of Pregnancy*,
https://doi.org/10.1007/978-3-030-49285-4_2

Epidemiology

PEP is the second most common dermatosis of pregnancy, with an incidence of 0.25–1.5% of all pregnancies [3–10]. Rates are significantly higher in multiple gestation pregnancies, affecting approximately 1 in 34 twin and 1 in 7 triplet pregnancies [11]. Overall, 2–16% of cases of PEP occur in multifetal pregnancies [5, 9, 10, 12–17]. While in vitro fertilization was used in many of the documented cases of PEP in multiple gestation pregnancies, a definite association has not been identified [7, 11].

Most reported cases of PEP are in white women [12, 18]. Patients are typically nulliparous (55–89%) and primigravidas (40–87%) [2, 5, 10, 12–17, 19, 20]. Many of the reported cases in multiparous and multigravid women occurred during their first multiple gestation pregnancy [6, 14, 21]. Some studies have shown skewed male:female ratios in offspring of patients with PEP, but this has been inconsistent [5, 16, 19].

Pathogenesis

Despite the prevalence of PEP, its etiology is poorly understood. Early literature suggested that PEP may be the pre-bullous phase of pemphigoid gestationis (PG); however, this theory has since been discredited [21]. Because PEP tends to arise in primigravidas within striae distensae and has a predilection for multiple gestation pregnancies, investigators have sought a correlation between maternal weight gain and PEP. However, observational studies have yielded mixed results [5, 10, 13, 18, 19]. Mechanical stress from abdominal weight gain may damage connective tissue in the striae, exposing an unidentified antigen in the skin and producing an immune-mediated inflammatory response [21–23]. Increased numbers of antigen presenting cells and Th lymphocytes have been identified in lesional tissue of patients with PEP, supporting an antigenic trigger [24]. The predilection for first pregnancies may be explained in part by an increased likelihood of striae in primigravid women and the development of immune tolerance in subsequent pregnancies [2, 22].

Fetal deoxyribonucleic acid (DNA) may also act as an antigenic trigger. Circulating fetal DNA increases in prevalence throughout pregnancy and is found in >90% of expectant mothers by the late third trimester [25]. Increased vascular permeability in the gravid abdominal skin may lead to deposition of chimeric cells and a subsequent immune response, in a manner paralleling graft-versus-host-disease [25, 26]. This theory is supported by a skewed CD4:CD8 profile and deposition of interferon-gamma and interleukin-2 in lesional skin [27].

Various hormonal fluctuations during pregnancy may also influence the development of PEP. Suprabasal keratinocytes from lesional skin of patients with PEP have increased expression of progesterone receptors when compared to nonlesional skin and controls [28]. Multiple gestation pregnancies may result in even higher circulating levels of progesterone, amplifying the rates of PEP in these patients [22]. Although one early study showed reduced levels of serum cortisol in PEP patients, these findings have not been replicated [16].

Intradermal eosinophils may play a pathologic role in the development of PEP [29]. Increased rates of atopy have been reported in some studies [15, 18]. Whether this represents overlap with atopic eruption of pregnancy or a true association between PEP and atopy remains to be determined.

Clinical Presentation

PEP typically presents late in pregnancy, with 75–94% of patients presenting in the third trimester [5, 9, 12–19, 27, 30] and 4–15% presenting in the immediate postpartum period [5, 13, 16–18, 20]. Among women presenting after delivery, the vast majority develop symptoms in the first 1–2 weeks postpartum [18]. Infrequently, women may present in the earlier two trimesters. Earlier presentation is more commonly associated with multiple gestation pregnancies and atypical clinical phenotypes [11, 15].

Classically, patients develop papules and wheals initially on the abdomen, arising within the striae distensae [1, 18, 31] (Fig. 2.1). Rapid centrifugal spread to the remainder of the trunk, buttocks, and proximal extremities is common. Less frequently, the eruption begins on the extensor surfaces of the limbs and rarely is isolated to the extremities without involvement of the trunk [18, 19]. Involvement of the umbilicus is rare, which can be helpful in differentiating PEP from PG [16, 17, 32]. Similarly, involvement of the face, palms and soles is uncommon in PEP [13, 15, 17, 18, 21, 32–34]. Mucosal involvement has not been reported.

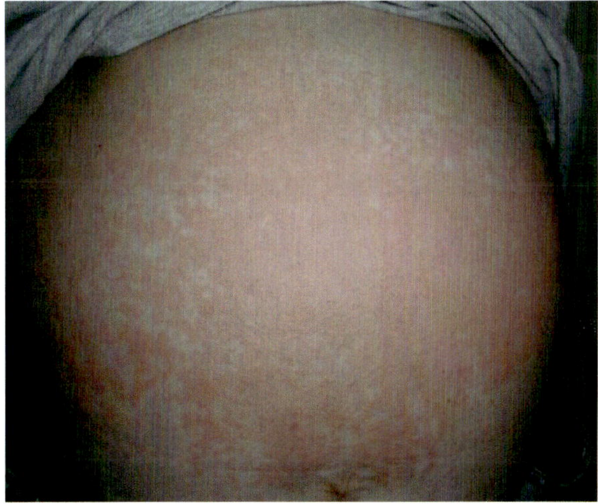

Fig. 2.1 Diffuse red patches and urticarial plaques on a gravid abdomen in a patient with PEP. (Courtesy of Dr. Steven Helms)

The most common morphology is intensely pruritic urticarial papules and plaques within striae. However, over half of patients may exhibit polymorphic features at some point during the course of the eruption, including polycyclic wheals, targetoid lesions, eczematous patches, blanching erythema, and vesicles [2, 15, 17–19]. Overt bullae are only rarely observed, in contrast to PG [35]. Patients with multifetal pregnancies may experience more severe symptoms [36].

In the absence of treatment, skin lesions tend to persist for approximately 6 weeks prior to spontaneous resolution, although the severity of symptoms frequently subsides after 1 week [18, 23]. Typically, delivery prompts resolution of symptoms over the course of several weeks [18]. Unlike PG, PEP does not flare in the immediate postpartum period [2]. Skin lesions may resolve with post-inflammatory hyperpigmentation [10].

Maternal and fetal outcomes are generally good in patients with PEP. Despite a possible association with increased maternal weight gain, a large observational study showed no significant increase in gestational diabetes [7]. One study suggested that hypertensive disorders and induction of labor may be more common in women with PEP [7]. It is unclear if PEP itself is an independent risk factor for caesarean section, as other risk factors including multifetal gestations and increased maternal weight gain need to be considered [7, 10, 12, 19]. Although infants born to mothers with PEP showed lower 5-minute Apgar scores, 1-minute Apgar scores were not significantly different from controls, and there was no significant difference in perinatal mortality (4.8% vs 1.5%, OR 3.3 [95% CI 0.8–13.8]) [7]. Spontaneous abortions and stillbirths have been reported in the fetuses of patients with PEP [5, 15, 16, 18], but no controlled cohorts have demonstrated a higher frequency than the general population.

Recurrence of PEP in subsequent pregnancies has rarely been reported, and recurrences may be less severe than the primary eruption [10, 17, 23, 37]. PEP does not flare with postpartum menstruation or the use of exogenous hormones, such as oral contraceptives [12, 23].

Pathology

The histopathology of PEP is nonspecific. Epidermal changes may be observed in approximately half of cases and include acanthosis, orthokeratosis, focal parakeratosis, and spongiosis [1, 2, 9, 13, 15, 16, 18, 31, 38]. Vesicles tend to be intraepidermal when present but may occasionally be subepidermal [6, 38]. A mild to moderate superficial and deep chronic perivascular infiltrate composed of lymphocytes, histiocytes, and a variable number of eosinophils is observed. Papillary dermal edema is common (Fig. 2.2).

Direct immunofluorescence (DIF) is negative or nonspecific and may differentiate PEP from PG. Sparse deposition of Complement factor 3 (C3), Immunoglobulin

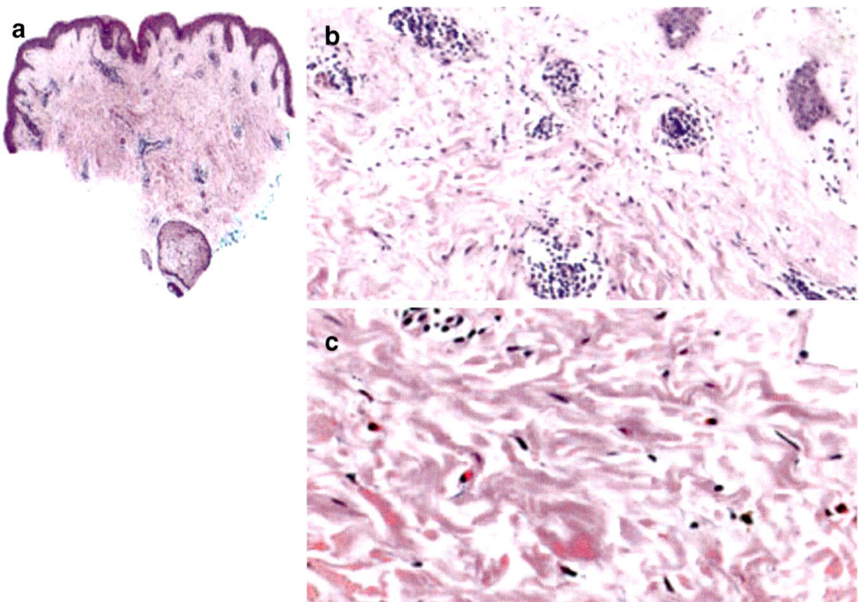

Fig. 2.2 Low power magnification shows perivascular inflammatory infiltrate with minimal changes in the epidermis (**a**, H&E 4×). The inflammatory infiltrate is mostly comprised of lymphocytes in a perivascular distribution with mild edema (**b**, H&E 20×). Eosinophils can be seen in some cases (**c**, H&E 40×). (Courtesy of Dr. Rami Al-Rohil, MD)

(Ig)M and IgA may be observed perivascularly and along the dermoepidermal junction [12, 15–18, 20, 39]. Indirect immunofluorescence (IIF) is negative.

Differential Diagnosis

PEP must be differentiated from other specific dermatoses of pregnancy, in particular from pemphigoid gestationis, which has different prognostic implications for the mother and fetus. PG shares many clinical features with PEP, including timing of onset, anatomic location, intense pruritis, and urticarial morphology. Sparing of the umbilicus and lesions arising within the striae distensae favors PEP over PG [2, 16, 17]. Skin biopsy cannot reliably distinguish PEP from PG, but DIF should demonstrate linear deposition of C3 and/or IgG at the dermoepidermal junction in PG [2]. IIF should have similar findings. If DIF was not performed at the time of biopsy and PEP and PG are both in the clinicopathologic differential diagnosis, immunohistochemical staining for C3d or C4d may be helpful in diagnosing PG [40, 41]. Additionally, enzyme-linked immunosorbent assays for the extracellular NC16a domain of BP-180 is a highly sensitive (96%) and specific (96%) diagnostic test for PG and should be negative in PEP [42].

The primary morphology of the lesions in specific cases of PEP may guide the differential diagnosis. Targetoid lesions must be distinguished from erythema multiforme, in particular EM driven by anogenital herpes simplex virus, which should be treated prior to vaginal delivery to prevent transmission to the fetus. Wheals should be differentiated from acute and chronic urticaria. Arthropod assault may present as papular urticaria. Acute urticaria may rarely be caused by anaphylaxis, which may be associated with maternal hypotension and shock and can have dire implications for the mother and fetus. Chronic urticaria may be associated with maternal hypothyroidism, which is imperative to treat intrapartum to prevent cognitive deficits in the offspring. Chronic urticaria may also be a manifestation of underlying infection or malignancy; in fact, a case of an urticarial eruption mimicking PEP in a patient with acute hepatitis B viral infection has been reported [43]. Eczematous lesions should be differentiated from atopic eruption of pregnancy. Like PEP, autoimmune progesterone dermatitis may be polymorphic with urticarial, papulovesicular, targetoid, or eczematous lesions, and a history of premenstrual flares of dermatitis or positive intradermal skin testing to progesterone can distinguish it from PEP [44].

Treatment

Management of patients with PEP is based primarily on the extent of the eruption and severity of symptoms. First line therapies include emollients, over-the-counter antipruritics such as menthol and urea, and mid- to high-potency topical corticosteroids [1, 12, 13, 18, 19, 31]. Oral antihistamines may be used as an adjuvant therapy for pruritis and insomnia [18, 19]. Occasionally, in severe cases, oral steroids may be required. Low doses of oral prednisone may be used and tapered over several weeks [12, 13, 36]. However, due to late pregnancy risks including premature delivery, premature rupture of membranes, and eclampsia, caution is advised, and the lowest effective dose should be used [45]. Use during breastfeeding is permitted, but mothers should be advised to attempt to time feedings 4 hours after the administration of systemic steroids to minimize steroid concentrations in breast milk [46]. In the absence of treatment, PEP will spontaneously resolve in the postpartum period [2].

Intramuscular injections of autologous whole blood have been proposed as an alternative to traditional therapies in women who are medication averse, based on reports of improvement in chronic urticaria and other dermatologic diseases [47, 48]. Of the few published cases where autologous whole blood injections were successfully used, three were in patients who presented earlier in the course of pregnancy than expected (14–28 weeks gestational age) [47], raising the possibility of an alternative diagnosis. One additional patient presented postpartum and experienced resolution several days after treatment was initiated [48], but it is difficult to determine whether the improvement can be attributed to the autologous whole blood injections, or whether this was the natural course of spontaneous resolution that is expected in the postpartum period. Further studies are required.

In rare refractory cases, early delivery may be necessary to alleviate PEP [36, 49].

Atopic Eruption of Pregnancy

Synonyms

Eczema of pregnancy; Prurigo gestationis (of Besnier); Prurigo of pregnancy; (Nurse's) Early onset prurigo of pregnancy; *Pruritic folliculitis of pregnancy; *Papular dermatitis of Spangler; *Linear IgM dermatosis of pregnancy.

Definition

Atopic eruption of pregnancy (AEP) is a relatively new term used to encompass multiple heterogeneous eczematous dermatoses arising in the context of pregnancy [17]. Historically, AEP has been separated into several other dermatoses, most notably eczema of pregnancy, prurigo of pregnancy, pruritic folliculitis of pregnancy, and papular dermatitis of Spangler. Distinguishing features of these entities have been inconsistent within the literature [17, 50]. Conflicting nomenclature and a lack of specific clinical or histologic elements have resulted in some controversy regarding classification [51, 52]. However, clinical and therapeutic overlap amongst the entities as well as a shared benign prognosis make AEP a useful unifying terminology.

Epidemiology

AEP is the most common pregnancy dermatosis, accounting for up to 50% of cases [17, 53, 54]. Prevalence ranges from 0.3% to 2% of all pregnancies [2, 55]. The vast majority of patients with AEP have an underlying atopic diathesis; 20–40% of women have a personal history of atopic dermatitis (AD), allergic rhinitis, or asthma [16, 17, 54], and an additional 50% have a family history of atopy [16]. Of note, the historic subclassifications pruritic folliculitis of pregnancy (PFP) and prurigo of pregnancy (PP) may not share an atopic association [50, 52].

---

*Some classifications group these entities with polymorphic eruption of pregnancy (PEP) or as separate dermatoses.

Pathogenesis

The exact mechanism of onset of the varied morphologies of AEP remains to be elucidated and is likely multifactorial. Mechanical stress on the skin during pregnancy may disrupt the skin barrier. Not surprisingly, women with filaggrin mutations are at increased risk for flares of AD during pregnancy [56].

During pregnancy, adaptive immunity shifts from Th1 to Th2 predominance, which is thought to prevent fetal rejection [57]. Subsequent increased production of IL-4 may contribute to elevations in serum immunoglobulin E (IgE) levels, a known manifestation of atopy. It has also been postulated that some skin manifestations classified as AEP may actually represent prurigo nodularis in patients with physiologic pruritis gravidarum and elevated IgE [16].

The high prevalence of AEP is likely driven by high overall rates of atopic dermatitis in the general population [58]. Undertreatment of pregnant patients, resulting from patient and physician reluctance to use topical and systemic medications, may contribute to flares in pregnancy.

Clinical Presentation

AEP is an umbrella diagnosis that embraces a clinically heterogeneous group of pruritic dermatoses arising during pregnancy. Compared to the other specific dermatoses of pregnancy, AEP has an earlier onset, with 50–75% of patients presenting in the first two trimesters [17, 53], and a mean onset of 18–22 weeks gestational age [17, 50]. AEP occurs in both primigravid and multigravid patients [17].

Ambros-Rudolph et al. [17] proposed stratifying AEP into E-type (eczematous) and P-type (papular) phenotypes.

E-type AEP includes exacerbations of pre-existing AD (20%) and new-onset eczematous eruptions (47%) (Fig. 2.3) [17]. Scaly erythematous thin plaques are observed predominantly either on the extremities or equally distributed on the trunk and extremities [17]. Although excoriations are common, primary skin lesions are mandatory for the diagnosis.

P-type AEP includes papular and folliculitic eruptions (31%) (Fig. 2.3) [17]. Although papular eczema falls into the P-type group, the association with underlying atopy in this subset is variable. Classically, the papular form of AEP has been called "[early-onset] prurigo of pregnancy" and "prurigo gestationis of Besnier." Individual lesions are small (<0.5 cm), erythematous, scaly papules on the arms and legs [50, 55] that may become lichenified, albeit usually to a lesser degree than typical prurigo nodularis of the nonpregnant patient [51]. The follicular form of P-type AEP is historically referred to as "pruritic folliculitis of pregnancy" (PFP). Both follicular-based inflammatory papules and acneiform pustules have been described [51, 59]. Unlike other forms of AEP, PFP may be minimally pruritic. In all varieties

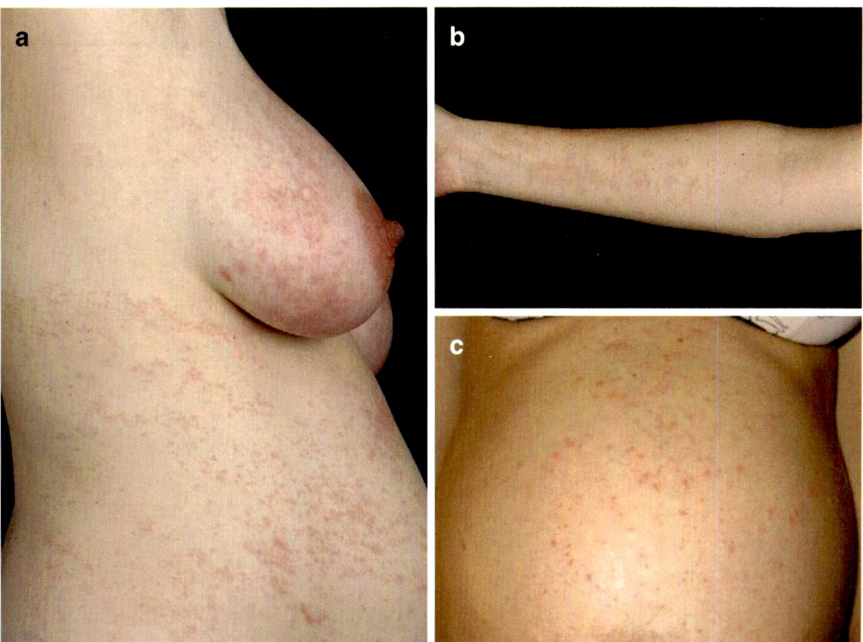

Fig. 2.3 Atopic eruption of pregnancy. E-type eczematous patches and plaques involving the trunk (**a**) and flexural extremities (**b**) in a 31-year-old primigravid woman. P-type erythematous papules clustered on the abdomen (**c**) in a 26-year-old primigravid woman. ((**a**, **b**) Reprinted with permission, Ambros-Rudolph et al. [17]. (**c**) Reprinted with permission, Roth [186])

of P-type AEP, excoriations are typical, and secondary crusting is common. Scarring secondary to manipulation of the lesions and resolution with post-inflammatory hyperpigmentation may occur [51].

Laboratory evaluation is largely unremarkable, with the exception of elevations in serum IgE in some patients [16, 17].

Although one early case series describing a widespread papular eruption of pregnancy reported poor fetal outcomes [60], similar data has not been reproduced, and the justifications driving the authors' conclusions have been questioned [2]. In general, all subtypes of AEP are thought to have a benign course for both the mother and child [16, 61, 62]. Although one study found a statistically significant association between maternal AD and premature rupture of the membranes, the absolute risk remained low, and there was no significant increased risk of fetal prematurity or stillbirth [58].

AEP tends to resolve 2–3 months after delivery, regardless of treatment [51]. However, as up to 40% of women have a personal history of atopic dermatitis, some patients will have flares of their pre-existing disease postpartum. Recurrence in future pregnancies is common [17, 50, 51, 53], possibly owing to the underlying atopic diathesis in many patients.

Pathology

The histopathology of AEP is nonspecific and variable [17, 63]. Specimens typically demonstrate epidermal acanthosis, hyperkeratosis, parakeratosis, and spongiosis. A mild to moderate perivascular lymphohistiocytic infiltrate admixed with eosinophils may be present. Less commonly, there is dermal edema and lymphocytic vasculitis. In cases of PFP, a sterile folliculitis may be observed. Direct and indirect immunofluorescence are characteristically negative [2, 17].

Differential Diagnosis

AEP should be distinguished from physiologic pruritis gravidarum, which presents without rash or with only secondary excoriations. Xerosis cutis may be observed during pregnancy and may produce diffuse fine scaling, especially on the lower extremities in the setting of peripheral edema, but it does not demonstrate true primary eczematous or papular lesions. It is important to distinguish AEP from the other specific dermatoses of pregnancy, including polymorphic eruption of pregnancy, intrahepatic cholestasis of pregnancy, and pemphigoid gestationis, which have important therapeutic and prognostic differences.

Autoimmune progesterone dermatitis is an entity that typically presents during the luteal phase of menstruation but has been reported to develop or worsen intrapartum [44]. The eruption may be polymorphic, demonstrating urticarial, erythema multiforme-like and eczematous lesions. A history of premenstrual flares of dermatitis or positive intradermal skin testing to progesterone can differentiate autoimmune progesterone dermatitis from AD and AEP.

Allergic and irritant contact dermatitis may be suspected based on the distribution of eczematous lesions and a history of inciting exposure.

Drug eruptions and infections, such as viral exanthems and pityriasis rosea, are also in the differential diagnosis of AEP. A morbiliform or papulosquamous morphology may distinguish these entities. Infestations such as scabies and other arthropod infections may demonstrate papular urticaria or burrows on exam.

A pre-existing diagnosis of AD or AEP does not preclude the development of a more consequential pregnancy dermatosis. An abrupt change in morphology or symptomatology should prompt re-evaluation of the diagnosis and management.

Treatment

Because the overall prognosis of AEP is benign, management is focused on alleviation of symptoms and avoidance of complications. Like atopic dermatitis, AEP may be complicated by superimposed infections such as impetigo and eczema herpeticum, which should be treated appropriately to reduce any potential risk to the mother and fetus.

First line topical therapies include emollients and over-the-counter anti-pruritics, such as menthol additives [17]. 3–10% urea cream may be helpful [17]. When required, the lowest effective potency nonhalogenated topical corticosteroid should be used [54, 64]. Use of super potent topical corticosteroids over large surface areas should be avoided, especially in the first trimester, due to the potential for systemic absorption and adverse fetal effects [54, 64].

Most systemic antihistamines may be used safely for pruritis in pregnancy. First generation antihistamines diphenhydramine and chlorpheniramine have demonstrated good safety profiles in pregnancy as have non-sedating second generation antihistamines such as cetirizine and loratadine [54].

Narrowband ultraviolet B phototherapy is also considered a safe and effective option in pregnancy [65]. Recent data suggests that folic acid should be supplemented in pregnant patients undergoing phototherapy [66].

For recalcitrant cases, short courses of oral steroids may be considered in the second and third trimesters. Use of systemic steroids in the first trimester is not recommended due to the potential risk of anatomic anomalies including cleft palate, and use in the later trimesters has been reported to increase the risk for intrauterine growth retardation [54, 64]. If necessary, systemic use of cyclosporine may be considered in close collaboration with the obstetrician due to potential risk of intrauterine growth retardation and maternal adverse events such as hypertension and nephrotoxicity [54].

Intrahepatic Cholestasis of Pregnancy

Synonyms

Cholestasis of pregnancy, cholestatic jaundice of pregnancy, obstetric cholestasis, icterus gravidarum, idiopathic jaundice of pregnancy, hepatosis of pregnancy, hepatotoxemia of pregnancy.

Definition

Intrahepatic cholestasis of pregnancy is the most common pregnancy-specific liver disease. It presents with reversible cholestasis associated with pregnancy and intense pruritus. It typically begins in the late second or third trimester of pregnancy and is associated with increased fetal risks including prematurity, stillbirth and fetal distress.

Epidemiology

The first description of intrahepatic cholestasis of pregnancy dates back to 1883 [67]. In the 1970s, incidences as high as 27% had been reported in specific geographical regions, primarily in Bolivia and Chile [68, 69]. However, there has been a marked reduction in disease within these areas with a prevalence now estimated to be between 1.5% and 4% [70]. The incidence in Europe, North America, Australia, and Asia remains low at less than 1% of all pregnancies [71–76]. In Chile and Scandinavia, there appears to be a temporal relation with increased disease incidence in the winter [72, 77]. Intrahepatic cholestasis of pregnancy is also more common in twin or multiple gestation pregnancies [78]. Other maternal risk factors associated with intrahepatic cholestasis of pregnancy include hepatitis C infection [79–81], advanced maternal age [82] and low levels of vitamin D [83] and selenium [84].

Pathogenesis

The pathogenesis of intrahepatic cholestasis of pregnancy is likely multifactorial with genetic, hormonal and environmental components playing a role [85].

Genetic ICP is common among first-degree relatives [86] and is clustered in various geographic regions. Mutations in two genes, *ABCB4* (ATP-binding cassette, subfamily B, member 4) [87] and *ABCB11 (*ATP binding cassette subfamily B, member 11) [88, 89] have been linked with ICP in up to 16% [93, 94] and 1% [95] of cases respectively. Both genes belong to the ATP binding cassette subfamily and are involved in hepatocellular transport and the bile salt export pump. Additional heterozygous genetic mutations have recently been identified in genes such as *ATP8B1*, *ABCC2*, and *TJP2* [90]. Further studies are needed to examine these potential causative mutations and to determine their true incidence within the patient population.

Hormonal Estrogen has been linked with ICP. In rat models, administration of estrogen will promote cholestasis through the impaired function of genes known to be related to the development of disease, including *ABCB11* and *ABCC2* [91, 92]. Estrogen has also been linked with cholestasis in women taking estrogen-containing contraceptives or hormone replacements [93]. Additionally, ICP typically presents at the end of pregnancy when estrogen levels are highest, and it is more common in multiple gestation pregnancies, which have higher levels of estrogen [78]. In addition to estrogen, progesterone has also been linked to ICP. Women treated early in their pregnancy with progesterone have an increased risk for ICP [94]. Furthermore, elevated levels of progesterone metabolites have been identified in the serum of affected females [95, 96]. The addition of these progesterone metabolites to in vitro experiments inhibited the bile salt export pump encoded by the gene *ABCB11*, which was previously found to carry mutations in patients with the disease [97].

Environmental Temporal trends in Chile and Scandinavia suggest an environmental influence [72, 77]. Low levels of vitamin D from decreased sunlight exposure [83] and low levels of selenium intake [77] are thought to contribute to this temporal trend [98]. Future studies will likely identify other environmental factors involved in the pathogenesis of intrahepatic cholestasis of pregnancy.

Clinical Presentation

ICP typically presents during the third trimester and has spontaneous resolution 1–2 weeks following delivery [99]. Unlike other dermatoses of pregnancy, intrahepatic cholestasis of pregnancy has no classic primary lesions. Severe pruritus occurs on the palms and soles, which then often generalizes to affect the entire body, especially the extremities, buttocks, and abdomen. Diffuse excoriations are seen on exam. Most patients experience worsening of pruritus at night, which may lead to insomnia [100]. Patients may also experience symptoms of cholestasis including jaundice, (often noticed 1–4 weeks following the onset of pruritus), anorexia, fatigue, dark urine and steatorrhea [101]. Symptoms resolve 1–2 weeks after delivery.

Diagnosis is confirmed by elevated levels of serum bile acids (>10 μmol/l in a pregnant woman). Liver function tests are also usually elevated. Rarely, the onset of pruritus can occur before biochemical changes [102].

Fetal morbidity can be significant with ICP, as damaging bile acids cross the placenta. Preterm delivery [103], spontaneous abortion [104], fetal distress [105] and meconium staining of amniotic fluid [103] have been associated with ICP. The high bile acids can affect cardiomyocytes causing fetal arrhythmias and can impose a vasoconstrictive effect on the placental chorionic veins leading to fetal distress, asphyxia, and fetal death [106, 107]. Additionally, the bile acids may affect the oxytocin receptors which may contribute to preterm labor [108].

The severity of complications correlates with the level of bile acids, with the most severe complications seen with the highest levels of bile acids [109]. Potential long-term sequelae for children born from mothers affected by ICP include increased fasting insulin levels, lower HDL, and higher BMIs [110].

Mothers affected by ICP were found to have a higher incidence of hepatitis C, nonalcoholic cirrhosis, gallstones and cholecystitis post-partum [111], although a direct cause and effect is difficult to discern.

Pathology

Histopathology of the skin reveals changes resulting from pruritus and exocoriation. Liver histopathology reveals acinar cholestasis with bile back-up into the canaliculi and hepatocytes. The bile ducts are relatively preserved, and there is limited inflammation apparent within the liver microstructure [112].

Differential Diagnosis

ICP should be distinguished from other dermatoses of pregnancy such as atopic eruption of pregnancy (AEP), polymorphic eruption of pregnancy (PEP) and pemphigoid gestationis (PG). Absence of specific skin findings and elevations of serum bile acids can assist with distinguishing ICP from these other dermatoses of pregnancy.

Viral hepatitis should be ruled out with viral serologies. Other liver conditions such as biliary obstruction, alcohol or drug-induced hepatitis, and HELLP (hemolysis, elevated liver enzymes, and low platelets) also need to be ruled out with an appropriate history and laboratory work-up.

Treatment

The mainstay of treatment for intrahepatic cholestasis of pregnancy is ursodeoxycholic acid. This treatment can be initiated empirically after the onset of pruritus [113, 114] or delayed until the first signs of bile acid elevation. Dosing is generally started at 300 mg two to three times a day [115] and is usually well-tolerated. Pruritus generally improves within 2 weeks, and serum bile acid and transaminase levels generally decline by 4 weeks [116]. If symptoms remain severe after 2 weeks, the medication can be increased weekly until either asymptomatic improvement is noted or a maximum dose of 21 mg/kg/day is achieved [114, 117]. Unfortunately, although ursodeoxycholic acid decreases maternal pruritus, a large randomized, controlled trial demonstrated that it does not reduce adverse perinatal outcomes [118].

If symptoms remain severe, additional medications can be utilized including cholestyramine [119, 120], rifampin [121, 122] or s-adenosyl-methionine [123]. Hydroxyzine and chlorpheniramine may also provide mild relief of pruritus.

Early delivery may be indicated to prevent fetal morbidity and mortality as well as provide maternal symptom relief. One large, retrospective cohort recommended delivery at 36 weeks gestation to reduce perinatal mortality [124], although this remains controversial. Regardless, the risk and benefits of early delivery must be considered, especially in the setting of significantly elevated serum bile acid levels [125].

Mothers must also be counseled that ICP can recur in up to 60–70% of future pregnancies. Additionally, medications containing high doses of estrogen, such as certain oral contraceptives, should be avoided to prevent disease flares.

Pemphigoid Gestationis

Synonyms

Gestational pemphigoid; herpes gestationis.

Definition

Pemphigoid gestationis is a rare autoimmune skin disorder presenting with intense pruritus and urticarial lesions that can progress to vesicular lesions, most frequently during the 2nd or 3rd trimester.

Epidemiology

The incidence of pemphigoid gestationis is estimated to be around 1 in 50,000–60,000 pregnancies in the United States [126, 127] and has been reported in similar incidences of 1 in 40,000 pregnancies in the UK [128, 129] and 1 in 7000 pregnancies in Switzerland [130]. In a majority of cases, the initial eruption begins in the 2nd or 3rd trimester with spontaneous resolution following delivery [131]. Rarely, the onset of pemphigoid gestationis is associated with hydatidiform moles or choriocarcinoma [132–134].

Pathogenesis

Pemphigoid gestationis is caused by autoantibodies to the noncollagenous domain (NC16A) of BP180. There is a strong association with major histocompatibility complex proteins Human Leukocyte Antigen (HLA)-DR3 and HLA-DR4. In one study from the United States, 61% of patients expressed HLA-DR3, 52% expressed HLA-DR4, and 43% of patients expressed a combination of HLA-DR3 and HLA-DR4 [135]. This association with Major Histocompatibility Complex (MHC) II molecules appears to be consistent across other ethnic groups including pregnant females from Mexico (HLA-DR3/HLA-DR4) [136] and Kuwait (HLA-DR2/HLA-DQ2) [137]. Aberrant expression of these MHCII molecules on placental tissues is thought to lead to the loss of immunotolerance of the placenta and fetus allowing for the uptake and processing of placental proteins including Bullous Pemphigoid (BP)180 [138]. BP180 is a hemidesmosomal protein [139] found in the amniotic epithelium and umbilical cord of the fetus as well as the skin of the mother [140, 141]. This loss of maternal-fetal immunotolerance allows for the development of autoantibodies against the NC16A domain of BP 180 [42, 142]. Although initially thought to belong to the IgG1 and IgG3 subclass of antibodies [146, 149], it is now believed that the predominant subclass is IgG4 [150], which is the subclass that crosses the placenta. This binding, in turn, activates the classical complement pathway resulting in immune cell infiltration [143]. Over 90% of PG patients also carry a C4 null allele causing a faulty complement system that impairs immune complex removal [144]. This immune cell activation and infiltration, especially of eosinophils [145], is thought to be the primary contributor to the disruption of the dermal-epidermal junction causing blister formation [146–148].

In addition to antibody production, alterations in female hormone levels during pregnancy likely contribute to the disease course. Estrogen is known to rise throughout pregnancy and increases the production of antibodies, the key mediators of pemphigoid gestationis. Conversely, progesterone, which decreases antibody production, peaks right before delivery and rapidly decreases postpartum, which may help explain flares of PG shortly after delivery [149, 150]. Changes in hormone levels are also implicated in disease flares during menstruation and oral contraceptive use [126, 131].

Clinical Presentation

Pemphigoid gestationis classically occurs during the second or third trimester. It usually begins with intense pruritus followed by the development of urticarial papules and plaques. In 90% of patients, the papules and plaques are initially located in the periumbilical area [131, 151, 152], but with time they will spread centrifugally to involve other cutaneous surfaces of the abdomen and the extremities, including the palms and soles (Fig. 2.4). Mucous membranes and the face are usually spared. The urticarial plaques can further progress to vesicles and tense vesicles or bullae in some patients [126, 153, 154]. Patients may experience a decrease in symptoms a few weeks before delivery, followed by a flare shortly after delivery. Following delivery, the urticarial plaques and vesicles or bullae will slowly subside with the majority of patients being symptom-free by 6 months [131]. There have been a few reports of subsequent development of bullous pemphigoid; however, this is uncommon [155].

Clinical findings in the fetus may be present upon delivery because of the transmission of autoantibodies across the placenta. Neonates have skin lesions approximately 5–10% of the time. Fortunately, skin findings in the neonate are usually mild urticarial papules and plaques and spontaneously resolve within days to weeks after delivery [156, 157]. PG is also associated with prematurity and small for gestational age infants, and these risks correlate with disease severity [158, 159].

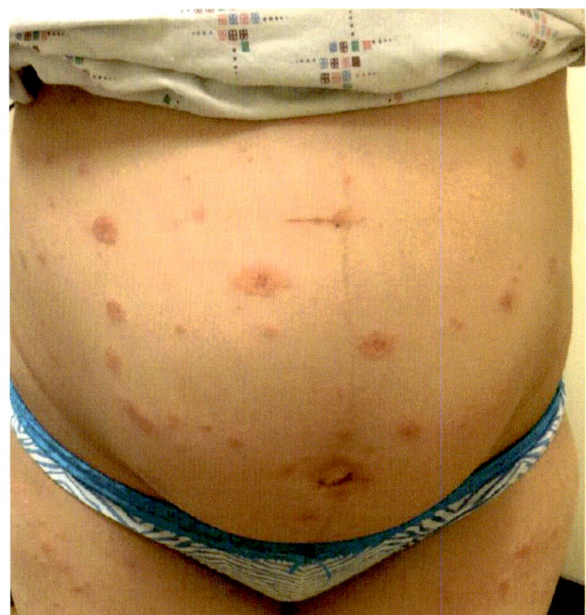

Fig. 2.4 Large urticarial plaques, including periumbical plaques, covering a gravid abdomen in a patient with PG

The risk of recurrence in future pregnancies is high and ranges from 33% to 50%. In multiparous women with a history of pemphigoid gestationis, recurrence has been associated with more severe disease and earlier onset during subsequent gestations [151]. Skip pregnancies may also be seen and occur in about 8% of patients [131], perhaps because of the full compatibility of fetus and mother during unaffected gestations.

Females with a history of pemphigoid gestationis have an increased risk for the development of Grave's disease when compared to the normal population [131], and family members of patients with pemphigoid gestationis have an increased risk of other autoimmune diseases [160]. This relationship to other autoimmune diseases is likely secondary to the presence of HLA-DR3 and HLA-DR4, which are involved in the development of autoimmunity.

Pathology

On histopathology, eosinophilic spongiosis with progression to a subepidermal blister with intralesional eosinophils is classically seen [161]. With direct immunofluorescence, complement 3 can be visualized in linear deposits along the basement membrane in the presence or absence of IgG [161]. These linear deposits bind to the epidermal side of salt-split skin testing. Enzyme-linked immunoassays (ELISAs) are also utilized and measure the presence of BP180 in maternal serum. Levels of the antibody can also be followed throughout the pregnancy and during treatment, as they correlate with disease severity [42, 162, 163]. The sensitivity and specificity of these tests are greater than 95% [42, 142, 147] and therefore, in the presence of classic skin findings, ELISA for BP180 may allow for a diagnosis without histopathology.

Differential Diagnosis

PG must be differentiated from other dermatoses of pregnancy, especially atopic eruption of pregnancy, polymorphic eruption of pregnancy (PEP), and intrahepatic cholestasis of pregnancy [139]. PEP shares many clinical features with PG including onset in late pregnancy, the involvement of the abdomen, intense pruritus, and urticarial plaques. However, the involvement of the umbilicus and the presence of blisters should help to differentiate PG from PEP. Furthermore, DIF findings of C3 and/or IgG at the dermo-epidermal junction and positive ELISA for BP180 should confirm a diagnosis of PG over PEP.

Other non-pregnancy related conditions must also be excluded including dermatitis herpetiformis, allergic contact dermatitis, and drug eruption [146]. Key defining features and histopathology with characteristic immunofluorescence findings are vital for appropriate diagnosis and treatment of pemphigoid gestationis.

Treatment

Management of PG is based on the extent of eruption and the severity of symptoms. Mild disease consisting of a few, localized lesions can be treated with mid to high potency topical steroids. For symptomatic control of the pruritus and insomnia, oral antihistamines can be added [146]. If symptoms remain uncontrolled, therapy may be escalated to oral corticosteroids, most commonly prednisone or prednisolone (up to 1 mg/kg/day) until symptoms are adequately managed [164]. After symptoms have stabilized, efforts to taper or discontinue oral corticosteroids should be considered in an effort to minimize risks, including premature delivery, premature rupture of membranes, and eclampsia [165, 166]. Intravenous immunoglobulin [167, 168], azathioprine [169], plasmapheresis/plasma exchange [170, 171], and cyclosporine [172] have been used during pregnancy in recalcitrant cases. Additionally, a case of successful use of rituximab during pregnancy in a recalcitrant PG patient has been published [184]. Persistent severe postpartum cases of PG have been treated with azathioprine [168], cyclosporine [173–175], cyclophosphamide [176], tetracyclines and nicotinamide [177, 178], dapsone [179], rituximab [180], plasmapheresis [170],and intravenous immunoglobulin [175, 181–185].

References

1. Lawley TJ, Hertz KC, Wade TR, Ackerman AB, Katz SI. Pruritic urticarial papules and plaques of pregnancy. J Am Med Assoc. 1979;241(16):1696–9.
2. Charles Holmes R, Black MM. The specific dermatoses of pregnancy. J Am Acad Dermatol. 1983;8(3):405–12.
3. Black MM. Refinements of the classification of polymorphic eruption of pregnancy. J Am Acad Dermatol. 2008;59(4):722–3.
4. Roger D, Vaillant L, Fignon A, Pierre F, Bacq Y, Brechot JF, Grangeponte MC, Lorette G. Specific pruritic diseases of pregnancy a prospective study of 3192 pregnant women. Arch Dermatol. 1994;130(6):734–9.
5. Regnier S, Fermand V, Levy P, Uzan S, Aractingi S. A case-control study of polymorphic eruption of pregnancy. J Am Acad Dermatol. 2008;58(1):63–7.
6. Holmes RC, McGibbon DH, Black MM. Polymorphic eruption of pregnancy with subepidermal vesicles. J R Soc Med. 1984;77(Suppl 4):22–3.
7. Ohel I, Levy A, Silberstein T, Holcberg G, Sheiner E. Pregnancy outcome of patients with pruritic urticarial papules and plaques of pregnancy. J Matern Fetal Neonatal Med. 2006;19(5):305–8.
8. Masood S, Rizvi DA, Tabassum S, Akhtar S, Alvi RU. Frequency and clinical variants of specific dermatoses in third trimester of pregnancy: a study from a tertiary care centre. J Pak Med Assoc. 2012;62(3):244–8.
9. Noguera J, Moreno A, Moragas JM. Pruritic urticarial papules and plaques of pregnancy (PUPPP). Acta Derm Venereol. 1983;63(1):35–8.
10. Bourne G. Toxaemic rash of pregnancy. Proc R Soc Med. 1962;55:462–4.
11. Elling SV, McKenna P, Powell FC. Pruritic urticarial papules and plaques of pregnancy in twin and triplet pregnancies. J Eur Acad Dermatol Venereol. 2000;14(5):378–81.
12. Yancey KB, Hall RP, Lawley TJ. Pruritic urticarial papules and plaques of pregnancy. Clinical experience in twenty-five patients. J Am Acad Dermatol. 1984;10(3):473–80.
13. Cohen LM, Capeless EL, Krusinski PA, Maloney ME. Pruritic urticarial papules and plaques of pregnancy and its relationship to maternal-fetal weight gain and twin pregnancy. Arch Dermatol. 1989;125(11):1534–6.
14. Powell FC. Parity, polypregnancy, paternity, and PUPPP. Arch Dermatol. 1992;128(11):1551.
15. Aronson IK, Bond S, Fiedler VC, Vomvouras S, Gruber D, Ruiz C. Pruritic urticarial papules and plaques of pregnancy: clinical and immunopathologic observations in 57 patients. J Am Acad Dermatol. 1998;39(6):933–9.
16. Vaughan Jones SA, Hern S, Nelson-Piercy C, Seed PT, Black MM. A prospective study of 200 women with dermatoses of pregnancy correlating clinical findings with hormonal and immunopathological profiles. Br J Dermatol. 1999;141(1):71–81.
17. Ambros-Rudolph CM, Müllegger RR, Vaughan-Jones SA, Kerl H, Black MM. The specific dermatoses of pregnancy revisited and reclassified: results of a retrospective two-center study on 505 pregnant patients. J Am Acad Dermatol. 2006;54(3):395–404.
18. Rudolph CM, Al-Fares S, Vaughan-Jones SA, Müllegger RR, Kerl H, Black MM. Polymorphic eruption of pregnancy: clinicopathology and potential trigger factors in 181 patients. Br J Dermatol. 2006;154(1):54–60.
19. Ghazeeri G, Kibbi AG, Abbas O. Pruritic urticarial papules and plaques of pregnancy: epidemiological, clinical, and histopathological study of 18 cases from Lebanon. Int J Dermatol. 2012;51(9):1047–53.
20. Alcalay J, Ingber A, David M, Hazaz B, Sandbank M. Pruritic urticarial papules and plaques of pregnancy. A review of 21 cases. J Reprod Med. 1987;32(4):315–6.

21. Vaughan Jones SA, Dunnill MG, Black MM. Pruritic urticarial papules and plaques of pregnancy (polymorphic eruption of pregnancy): two unusual cases. Br J Dermatol. 1996;135(1):102–5.
22. Ahmadi S, Powell FC. Pruritic urticarial papules and plaques of pregnancy: current status. Australas J Dermatol. 2005;46(2):53–8; quiz 59.
23. Charles-Holmes R. Polymorphic eruption of pregnancy. Semin Dermatol. 1989;8(1):18–22.
24. Carli P, Tarocchi S, Mello G, Fabbri P. Skin immune system activation in pruritic urticarial papules and plaques of pregnancy. Int J Dermatol. 1994;33(12):884–5.
25. Aractingi S, Berkane N, Bertheau P, le Goué C, Dausset J, Uzan S, et al. Fetal DNA in skin of polymorphic eruptions of pregnancy. Lancet. 1998;352(9144):1898–901.
26. Kroumpouzos G, Cohen LM. Specific dermatoses of pregnancy: an evidence-based systematic review. Am J Obstet Gynecol. 2003;188(4):1083–92.
27. Caproni M, Giomi B, Berti S, Bianchi B, Fabbri P. Relevance of cellular infiltrate and cytokines in polymorphic eruption of pregnancy (PEP). J Dermatol Sci. 2006;43(1):67–9.
28. Im S, Lee ES, Kim W, Song J, Kim J, Lee M, et al. Expression of progesterone receptor in human keratinocytes. J Korean Med Sci. 2000;15(6):647–54.
29. Borrego L, Peterson EA, Diez LI, de Pablo Martin P, Wagner JM, Gleich GJ, et al. Polymorphic eruption of pregnancy and herpes gestationis: comparison of granulated cell proteins in tissue and serum. Clin Exp Dermatol. 1999;24(3):213–25.
30. Alcalay J, Ingber A, Hazaz B, David M, Sandbank M. Linear IgM dermatosis of pregnancy. J Am Acad Dermatol. 1988;18(2 Pt 2):412–5.
31. Callen JP, Hanno R. Pruritic urticarial papules and plaques of pregnancy (PUPPP). A clinicopathologic study. J Am Acad Dermatol. 1981;5(4):401–5.
32. Kirkup ME, Dunnill MGS. Polymorphic eruption of pregnancy developing in the puerperium. Clin Exp Dermatol. 2002;27(8):657–60.
33. Özcan D, Özçakmak B, Aydoğan FÇ. Polymorphic eruption of pregnancy with palmoplantar involvement that developed after delivery. J Obstet Gynaecol Res. 2011;37(8):1158–61.
34. High WA, Hoang MP, Miller MD. Pruritic urticarial papules and plaques of pregnancy with unusual and extensive palmoplantar involvement. Obstet Gynecol. 2005;105(5 II):1261–4.
35. Sherley-Dale AC, Carr RA, Charles-Holmes R. Polymorphic eruption of pregnancy with bullous lesions: a previously unreported association. Br J Dermatol. 2010;162(1):220–2.
36. Bunker CB, Erskine K, Rustin MH, Gilkes JJ. Severe polymorphic eruption of pregnancy occurring in twin pregnancies. Clin Exp Dermatol. 1990;15(3):228–31.
37. Patel P, Ashack KA, Aronson IK. Postpartum polymorphic eruption of pregnancy: an unusual presentation. Int J Dermatol. 2019;58(3):357–9.
38. Moreno A, Noguera J, de Moragas JM. Polymorphic eruption of pregnancy: histopathologic study. Acta Derm Venereol. 1985;65(4):313–8.
39. Tarocchi S, Carli P, Caproni M, Fabbri P. Polymorphic eruption of pregnancy. Int J Dermatol. 1997;36(6):448–50.
40. Kwon EJ, Ntiamoah P, Shulman KJ. The utility of C4d immunohistochemistry on formalin-fixed paraffin-embedded tissue in the distinction of polymorphic eruption of pregnancy from pemphigoid gestationis. Am J Dermatopathol. 2013;35(8):787–91.
41. Pfaltz K, Mertz K, Rose C, Scheidegger P, Pfaltz M, Kempf W. C3d immunohistochemistry on formalin-fixed tissue is a valuable tool in the diagnosis of bullous pemphigoid of the skin. J Cutan Pathol. 2010;37(6):654–8.
42. Powell AM, Sakuma-Oyama Y, Oyama N, Albert S, Bhogal B, Kaneko F, et al. Usefulness of BP180 NC16a enzyme-linked immunosorbent assay in the serodiagnosis of pemphigoid gestationis and in differentiating between pemphigoid gestationis and pruritic urticarial papules and plaques of pregnancy. Arch Dermatol. 2005;141(6):705–10.
43. Lozano-Masdemont B, Gómez-Recuero-Muñoz L, Pulido-Pérez A, Molina-López I, Suárez-Fernández R. Urticarial exanthema due to hepatitis B in a pregnant woman, mimicking a polymorphic eruption of pregnancy. Clin Exp Dermatol. 2016;41(8):896–8.
44. Herzberg AJ, Strohmeyer CR, Cirillo-Hyland VA. Autoimmune progesterone dermatitis. J Am Acad Dermatol. 1995;32(2 Pt 2):333–8.

45. Murase JE, Heller MM, Butler DC. Safety of dermatologic medications in pregnancy and lactation: part I. Pregnancy. J Am Acad Dermatol. 2014;70(3):401.e1–14; quiz 415.
46. Butler DC, Heller MM, Murase JE. Safety of dermatologic medications in pregnancy and lactation Part II. Lactation. J Am Acad Dermatol. 2014;70(3):417.e1–10; quiz 427.
47. Jeon IK, On HR, Oh SH, Hann SK. Three cases of pruritic urticarial papules and plaques of pregnancy (PUPPP) treated with intramuscular injection of autologous whole blood. J Eur Acad Dermatol Venereol. 2015;29(4):797–800.
48. Kim EH. Pruritic urticarial papules and plaques of pregnancy occurring postpartum treated with intramuscular injection of autologous whole blood. Case Rep Dermatol. 2017;9(1):151–6.
49. Beltrani VP, Beltrani VS. Pruritic urticarial papules and plaques of pregnancy: a severe case requiring early delivery for relief of symptoms. J Am Acad Dermatol. 1992;26(2):266–7.
50. Roger D, Vaillant L, Fignon A, Pierre F, Bacq Y, et al. Specific pruritic diseases of pregnancy a prospective study of 3192 pregnant women. Arch Dermatol. 1994;130(6):734–9.
51. Roth MM, Cristodor P, Kroumpouzos G. Prurigo, pruritic folliculitis, and atopic eruption of pregnancy: facts and controversies. Clin Dermatol. 2016;34(3):392–400.
52. Ingber A. Atopic eruption of pregnancy. J Eur Acad Dermatol Venereol. 2010;24(8):984.
53. Hassan I, Bashir S, Taing S. A clinical study of the skin changes in pregnancy in Kashmir valley of north India: a hospital based study. Indian J Dermatol. 2015;60(1):28–32.
54. Koutroulis I, Papoutsis J, Kroumpouzos G. Atopic dermatitis in pregnancy: current status and challenges. Obstet Gynecol Surv. 2011;66(10):654–63.
55. Nurse DS. Prurigo of pregnancy. Australas J Dermatol. 1968;9(3):258–67.
56. Bager P, Wohlfahrt J, Boyd H, Thyssen JP, Melbye M. The role of filaggrin mutations during pregnancy and postpartum: atopic dermatitis and genital skin diseases. Allergy: Eur J Allergy Clin Immunol. 2016;71(5):724–7.
57. Yang CS, Teeple M, Muglia J, Robinson-Bostom L. Inflammatory and glandular skin disease in pregnancy. Clin Dermatol. 2016;34(3):335–43.
58. Hamann CR, Egeberg A, Wollenberg A, Gislason G, Skov L, Thyssen JP. Pregnancy complications, treatment characteristics and birth outcomes in women with atopic dermatitis in Denmark. J Eur Acad Dermatol Venereol. 2019;33(3):577–87.
59. Zoberman E, Farmer ER. Pruritic folliculitis of pregnancy. Arch Dermatol. 1981;117(1):20–2.
60. Spangler AS, Reddy W, Bardawil WA, Roby CC, Emerson K. Papular dermatitis of pregnancy a new clinical entity? J Am Med Assoc. 1962;181:577–81.
61. Trønnes H, Wilcox AJ, Markestad T, Tollånes MC, Lie RT, Moster D. Associations of maternal atopic diseases with adverse pregnancy outcomes: a national cohort study. Paediatr Perinat Epidemiol. 2014;28(6):489–97.
62. Seeger JD, Lanza LL, West WA, Fernandez C, Rivero E. Pregnancy and pregnancy outcome among women with inflammatory skin diseases. Dermatology. 2006;214(1):32–9.
63. Massone C, Cerroni L, Heidrun N, Brunasso AMG, Nunzi E, Gulia A, et al. Histopathological diagnosis of atopic eruption of pregnancy and polymorphic eruption of pregnancy: a study on 41 cases. Am J Dermatopathol. 2014;36(10):812–21.
64. Chi C-C, Wang S-H, Wojnarowska F, Kirtschig G, Davies E, Bennett C. Safety of topical corticosteroids in pregnancy. Cochrane Database Syst Rev. 2015;(10):CD007346.
65. Roth M-M. Pregnancy dermatoses diagnosis, management, and controversies. Am J Clin Dermatol. 2011;12(1):25–41.
66. Park KK, Murase JE. Narrowband UV-B phototherapy during pregnancy and folic acid depletion. Arch Dermatol. 2012;148(1):132–3.
67. Pusl T, Beuers U. Intrahepatic cholestasis of pregnancy. Orphanet J Rare Dis. 2007;2:26.
68. Reyes H, Gonzalez MC, Ribalta J, Aburto H, Matus C, Schramm G, et al. Prevalence of intrahepatic cholestasis of pregnancy in Chile. Ann Intern Med. 1978;88(4):487–93.
69. Reyes H, Taboada G, Ribalta J. Prevalence of intrahepatic cholestasis of pregnancy in La Paz, Bolivia. J Chronic Dis. 1979;32(7):499–504.
70. Reyes H. Sex hormones and bile acids in intrahepatic cholestasis of pregnancy. Hepatology (Baltimore, MD). 2008;47(2):376–9.

71. Roncaglia N, Arreghini A, Locatelli A, Bellini P, Andreotti C, Ghidini A. Obstetric cholestasis: outcome with active management. Eur J Obstet Gynecol Reprod Biol. 2002;100(2):167–70.
72. Berg B, Helm G, Petersohn L, Tryding N. Cholestasis of pregnancy. Clinical and laboratory studies. Acta Obstet Gynecol Scand. 1986;65(2):107–13.
73. Laifer SA, Stiller RJ, Siddiqui DS, Dunston-Boone G, Whetham JC. Ursodeoxycholic acid for the treatment of intrahepatic cholestasis of pregnancy. J Matern Fetal Med. 2001;10(2):131–5.
74. Abedin P, Weaver JB, Egginton E. Intrahepatic cholestasis of pregnancy: prevalence and ethnic distribution. Ethn Health. 1999;4(1–2):35–7.
75. Lo TK, Lau WL, Lam HS, Leung WC, Chin RK. Obstetric cholestasis in Hong Kong--local experience with eight consecutive cases. Hong Kong Med J (Xianggang yi xue za zhi). 2007;13(5):387–91.
76. Gardiner FW, McCuaig R, Arthur C, Carins T, Morton A, Laurie J, et al. The prevalence and pregnancy outcomes of intrahepatic cholestasis of pregnancy: a retrospective clinical audit review. Obstet Med. 2019;12(3):123–8.
77. Reyes H, Báez ME, González MC, Hernández I, Palma J, Ribalta J, et al. Selenium, zinc and copper plasma levels in intrahepatic cholestasis of pregnancy, in normal pregnancies and in healthy individuals, in Chile. J Hepatol. 2000;32(4):542–9.
78. Gonzalez MC, Reyes H, Arrese M, Figueroa D, Lorca B, Andresen M, et al. Intrahepatic cholestasis of pregnancy in twin pregnancies. J Hepatol. 1989;9(1):84–90.
79. Wijarnpreecha K, Thongprayoon C, Sanguankeo A, Upala S, Ungprasert P, Cheungpasitporn W. Hepatitis C infection and intrahepatic cholestasis of pregnancy: a systematic review and meta-analysis. Clin Res Hepatol Gastroenterol. 2017;41(1):39–45.
80. Locatelli A, Roncaglia N, Arreghini A, Bellini P, Vergani P, Ghidini A. Hepatitis C virus infection is associated with a higher incidence of cholestasis of pregnancy. Br J Obstet Gynaecol. 1999;106(5):498–500.
81. Marschall HU, Wikstrom Shemer E, Ludvigsson JF, Stephansson O. Intrahepatic cholestasis of pregnancy and associated hepatobiliary disease: a population-based cohort study. Hepatology (Baltimore, MD). 2013;58(4):1385–91.
82. Heinonen S, Kirkinen P. Pregnancy outcome with intrahepatic cholestasis. Obstet Gynecol. 1999;94(2):189–93.
83. Wikstrom Shemer E, Marschall HU. Decreased 1,25-dihydroxy vitamin D levels in women with intrahepatic cholestasis of pregnancy. Acta Obstet Gynecol Scand. 2010;89(11):1420–3.
84. Kauppila A, Korpela H, Makila UM, Yrjanheikki E. Low serum selenium concentration and glutathione peroxidase activity in intrahepatic cholestasis of pregnancy. Br Med J (Clin Res Ed). 1987;294(6565):150–2.
85. Lammert F, Marschall H-U, Glantz A, Matern S. Intrahepatic cholestasis of pregnancy: molecular pathogenesis, diagnosis and management. J Hepatol. 2000;33(6):1012–21.
86. Turunen K, Helander K, Mattila KJ, Sumanen M. Intrahepatic cholestasis of pregnancy is common among patients' first-degree relatives. Acta Obstet Gynecol Scand. 2013;92(9):1108–10.
87. Dixon PH, Weerasekera N, Linton KJ, Donaldson O, Chambers J, Egginton E, et al. Heterozygous MDR3 missense mutation associated with intrahepatic cholestasis of pregnancy: evidence for a defect in protein trafficking. Hum Mol Genet. 2000;9(8):1209–17.
88. Dixon PH, Wadsworth CA, Chambers J, Donnelly J, Cooley S, Buckley R, et al. A comprehensive analysis of common genetic variation around six candidate loci for intrahepatic cholestasis of pregnancy. Am J Gastroenterol. 2014;109(1):76–84.
89. Anzivino C, Odoardi MR, Meschiari E, Baldelli E, Facchinetti F, Neri I, et al. ABCB4 and ABCB11 mutations in intrahepatic cholestasis of pregnancy in an Italian population. Dig Liver Dis. 2013;45(3):226–32.
90. Dixon PH, Sambrotta M, Chambers J, Taylor-Harris P, Syngelaki A, Nicolaides K, et al. An expanded role for heterozygous mutations of ABCB4, ABCB11, ATP8B1, ABCC2 and TJP2 in intrahepatic cholestasis of pregnancy. Sci Rep. 2017;7(1):11823.

91. Yamamoto Y, Moore R, Hess HA, Guo GL, Gonzalez FJ, Korach KS, et al. Estrogen receptor alpha mediates 17alpha-ethynylestradiol causing hepatotoxicity. J Biol Chem. 2006;281(24):16625–31.
92. Crocenzi FA, Mottino AD, Cao J, Veggi LM, Pozzi EJ, Vore M, et al. Estradiol-17beta-D-glucuronide induces endocytic internalization of Bsep in rats. Am J Physiol Gastrointest Liver Physiol. 2003;285(2):G449–59.
93. Dong R, Wang J, Gao X, Wang C, Liu K, Wu J, et al. Yangonin protects against estrogen-induced cholestasis in a farnesoid X receptor-dependent manner. Eur J Pharmacol. 2019;857:172461.
94. Bacq Y, Sapey T, Brechot MC, Pierre F, Fignon A, Dubois F. Intrahepatic cholestasis of pregnancy: a French prospective study. Hepatology (Baltimore, MD). 1997;26(2):358–64.
95. Reyes H, Sjövall J. Bile acids and progesterone metabolites intrahepatic cholestasis of pregnancy. Ann Med. 2000;32(2):94–106.
96. Meng L, Reyes H, Axelson M, Palma J, Hernandez I, Ribalta J, et al. Progesterone metabolites and bile acids in serum of patients with intrahepatic cholestasis of pregnancy: effect of ursodeoxycholic acid therapy. Hepatology (Baltimore, MD). 1997;26(6):1573–9.
97. Vallejo M, Briz O, Serrano MA, Monte MJ, Marin JJG. Potential role of trans-inhibition of the bile salt export pump by progesterone metabolites in the etiopathogenesis of intrahepatic cholestasis of pregnancy. J Hepatol. 2006;44(6):1150–7.
98. Floreani A, Gervasi MT. New insights on intrahepatic cholestasis of pregnancy. Clin Liver Dis. 2016;20(1):177–89.
99. Kenyon AP, Piercy CN, Girling J, Williamson C, Tribe RM, Shennan AH. Obstetric cholestasis, outcome with active management: a series of 70 cases. BJOG. 2002;109(3):282–8.
100. Geenes V, Williamson C. Intrahepatic cholestasis of pregnancy. World J Gastroenterol. 2009;15(17):2049–66.
101. Reyes H, Radrigan ME, Gonzalez MC, Latorre R, Ribalta J, Segovia N, et al. Steatorrhea in patients with intrahepatic cholestasis of pregnancy. Gastroenterology. 1987;93(3):584–90.
102. Kenyon AP, Piercy CN, Girling J, Williamson C, Tribe RM, Shennan AH. Pruritus may precede abnormal liver function tests in pregnant women with obstetric cholestasis: a longitudinal analysis. BJOG. 2001;108(11):1190–2.
103. Fisk NM, Storey GN. Fetal outcome in obstetric cholestasis. Br J Obstet Gynaecol. 1988;95(11):1137–43.
104. Reid R, Ivey KJ, Rencoret RH, Storey B. Fetal complications of obstetric cholestasis. Br Med J. 1976;1(6014):870–2.
105. Shaw D, Frohlich J, Wittmann BA, Willms M. A prospective study of 18 patients with cholestasis of pregnancy. Am J Obstet Gynecol. 1982;142(6 Pt 1):621–5.
106. Williamson C, Gorelik J, Eaton BM, Lab M, de Swiet M, Korchev Y. The bile acid taurocholate impairs rat cardiomyocyte function: a proposed mechanism for intra-uterine fetal death in obstetric cholestasis. Clin Sci (Lond, Engl: 1979). 2001;100(4):363–9.
107. Sepulveda WH, Gonzalez C, Cruz MA, Rudolph MI. Vasoconstrictive effect of bile acids on isolated human placental chorionic veins. Eur J Obstet Gynecol Reprod Biol. 1991;42(3):211–5.
108. Germain AM, Kato S, Carvajal JA, Valenzuela GJ, Valdes GL, Glasinovic JC. Bile acids increase response and expression of human myometrial oxytocin receptor. Am J Obstet Gynecol. 2003;189(2):577–82.
109. Glantz A, Marschall HU, Mattsson LA. Intrahepatic cholestasis of pregnancy: Relationships between bile acid levels and fetal complication rates. Hepatology (Baltimore, MD). 2004;40(2):467–74.
110. Papacleovoulou G, Abu-Hayyeh S, Nikolopoulou E, Briz O, Owen BM, Nikolova V, et al. Maternal cholestasis during pregnancy programs metabolic disease in offspring. J Clin Invest. 2013;123(7):3172–81.

111. Ropponen A, Sund R, Riikonen S, Ylikorkala O, Aittomaki K. Intrahepatic cholestasis of pregnancy as an indicator of liver and biliary diseases: a population-based study. Hepatology (Baltimore, MD). 2006;43(4):723–8.
112. Rolfes DB, Ishak KG. Liver disease in pregnancy. Histopathology. 1986;10(6):555–70.
113. Kremer AE, Oude Elferink RP, Beuers U. Pathophysiology and current management of pruritus in liver disease. Clin Res Hepatol Gastroenterol. 2011;35(2):89–97.
114. Bacq Y, le Besco M, Lecuyer AI, Gendrot C, Potin J, Andres CR, et al. Ursodeoxycholic acid therapy in intrahepatic cholestasis of pregnancy: results in real-world conditions and factors predictive of response to treatment. Dig Liver Dis. 2017;49(1):63–9.
115. Bicocca MJ, Sperling JD, Chauhan SP. Intrahepatic cholestasis of pregnancy: review of six national and regional guidelines. Eur J Obstet Gynecol Reprod Biol. 2018;231:180–7.
116. Williamson C, Geenes V. Intrahepatic cholestasis of pregnancy. Obstet Gynecol. 2014;124(1):120–33.
117. Mazzella G, Rizzo N, Azzaroli F, Simoni P, Bovicelli L, Miracolo A, et al. Ursodeoxycholic acid administration in patients with cholestasis of pregnancy: effects on primary bile acids in babies and mothers. Hepatology (Baltimore, MD). 2001;33(3):504–8.
118. Chappell LC, Bell JL, Smith A, Linsell L, Juszczak E, Dixon PH, et al. Ursodeoxycholic acid versus placebo in women with intrahepatic cholestasis of pregnancy (PITCHES): a randomised controlled trial. Lancet. 2019;394(10201):849–60.
119. Mela M, Mancuso A, Burroughs AK. Review article: pruritus in cholestatic and other liver diseases. Aliment Pharmacol Ther. 2003;17(7):857–70.
120. Kondrackiene J, Beuers U, Kupcinskas L. Efficacy and safety of ursodeoxycholic acid versus cholestyramine in intrahepatic cholestasis of pregnancy. Gastroenterology. 2005;129(3):894–901.
121. Liu J, Murray AM, Mankus EB, Ireland KE, Acosta OM, Ramsey PS. Adjuvant use of rifampin for refractory intrahepatic cholestasis of pregnancy. Obstet Gynecol. 2018;132(3):678–81.
122. Geenes V, Chambers J, Khurana R, Shemer EW, Sia W, Mandair D, et al. Rifampicin in the treatment of severe intrahepatic cholestasis of pregnancy. Eur J Obstet Gynecol Reprod Biol. 2015;189:59–63.
123. Zhang Y, Lu L, Victor DW, Xin Y, Xuan S. Ursodeoxycholic acid and S-adenosylmethionine for the treatment of intrahepatic cholestasis of pregnancy: a meta-analysis. Hepat Mon. 2016;16(8):e38558.
124. Puljic A, Kim E, Page J, Esakoff T, Shaffer B, LaCoursiere DY, et al. The risk of infant and fetal death by each additional week of expectant management in intrahepatic cholestasis of pregnancy by gestational age. Am J Obstet Gynecol. 2015;212(5):667. e1–5.
125. Ovadia C, Seed PT, Sklavounos A, Geenes V, Di Ilio C, Chambers J, et al. Association of adverse perinatal outcomes of intrahepatic cholestasis of pregnancy with biochemical markers: results of aggregate and individual patient data meta-analyses. Lancet (Lond, Engl). 2019;393(10174):899–909.
126. Shornick JK, Bangert JL, Freeman RG, Gilliam JN. Herpes gestationis: clinical and histologic features of twenty-eight cases. J Am Acad Dermatol. 1983;8(2):214–24.
127. Kolodny RC. Herpes gestationis. A new assessment of incidence, diagnosis, and fetal prognosis. Am J Obstet Gynecol. 1969;104(1):39–45.
128. Black MM. Progress and new directions in the investigation of the specific dermatoses of pregnancy. Keio J Med. 1997;46(1):40–1.
129. Holmes RC, Black MM, Dann J, James DC, Bhogal B. A comparative study of toxic erythema of pregnancy and herpes gestationis. Br J Dermatol. 1982;106(5):499–510.
130. Zurn A, Celebi CR, Bernard P, Didierjean L, Saurat JH. A prospective immunofluorescence study of 111 cases of pruritic dermatoses of pregnancy: IgM anti-basement membrane zone antibodies as a novel finding. Br J Dermatol. 1992;126(5):474–8.
131. Jenkins RE, Hern S, Black MM. Clinical features and management of 87 patients with pemphigoid gestationis. Clin Exp Dermatol. 1999;24(4):255–9.

132. Tillman WG. Herpes gestationis with hydatidiform mole and chorion epithelioma. Br Med J. 1950;1(4668):1471.
133. Slazinski L, Degefu S. Herpes gestationis associated with choriocarcinoma. Arch Dermatol. 1982;118(6):425–8.
134. Tindall JG, Rea TH, Shulman I, Quismorio FP Jr. Herpes gestationis in association with a hydatidiform mole. Immunopathologic studies. Arch Dermatol. 1981;117(8):510–2.
135. Shornick JK, Stastny P, Gilliam JN. High frequency of histocompatibility antigens HLA-DR3 and DR4 in herpes gestations. J Clin Invest. 1981;68(2):553–5.
136. Garcia-Gonzalez E, Castro-Llamas J, Karchmer S, Zuniga J, de Oca DM, Ambaz M, et al. Class II major histocompatibility complex typing across the ethnic barrier in pemphigoid gestationis. A study in Mexicans. Int J Dermatol. 1999;38(1):46–51.
137. Nanda A, Al-Saeed K, Dvorak R, Al-Muzairai I, Al-Sabah H, Al-Arbash M, et al. Clinicopathological features and HLA tissue typing in pemphigoid gestationis patients in Kuwait. Clin Exp Dermatol. 2003;28(3):301–6.
138. Sadik CD, Lima AL, Zillikens D. Pemphigoid gestationis: toward a better understanding of the etiopathogenesis. Clin Dermatol. 2016;34(3):378–82.
139. Huilaja L, Mäkikallio K, Tasanen K. Gestational pemphigoid. Orphanet J Rare Dis. 2014;9:136.
140. Fairley JA, Heintz PW, Neuburg M, Diaz LA, Giudice GJ. Expression pattern of the bullous pemphigoid-180 antigen in normal and neoplastic epithelia. Br J Dermatol. 1995;133(3):385–91.
141. Ortonne JP, Hsi BL, Verrando P, Bernerd F, Pautrat G, Pisani A, et al. Herpes gestationis factor reacts with the amniotic epithelial basement membrane. Br J Dermatol. 1987;117(2):147–54.
142. Al Saif F, Jouen F, Hebert V, Chiavelli H, Darwish B, Duvert-Lehembre S, et al. Sensitivity and specificity of BP180 NC16A enzyme-linked immunosorbent assay for the diagnosis of pemphigoid gestationis. J Am Acad Dermatol. 2017;76(3):560–2.
143. Carruthers JA, Ewins AR. Herpes gestationis: studies on the binding characteristics, activity and pathogenetic significance of the complement-fixing factor. Clin Exp Immunol. 1978;31(1):38–44.
144. Shornick JK, Artlett CM, Jenkins RE, Briggs DC, Welsh KI, Garvey MP, et al. Complement polymorphism in herpes gestationis: association with C4 null allele. J Am Acad Dermatol. 1993;29(4):545–9.
145. Scheman AJ, Hordinsky MD, Groth DW, Vercellotti GM, Leiferman KM. Evidence for eosinophil degranulation in the pathogenesis of herpes gestationis. Arch Dermatol. 1989;125(8):1079–83.
146. Kelly SE, et al. The distribution of IgG subclasses in pemphigoid gestationis: PG factor is an IgG1 autoantibody. J Invest Dermatol. 1989;92(5):695–8.
147. Sitaru C, Schmidt E, Petermann S, Munteanu LS, Brocker EB, Zillikens D. Autoantibodies to bullous pemphigoid antigen 180 induce dermal-epidermal separation in cryosections of human skin. J Invest Dermatol. 2002;118(4):664–71.
148. Shimanovich I, Mihai S, Oostingh GJ, Ilenchuk TT, Brocker EB, Opdenakker G, et al. Granulocyte-derived elastase and gelatinase B are required for dermal-epidermal separation induced by autoantibodies from patients with epidermolysis bullosa acquisita and bullous pemphigoid. J Pathol. 2004;204(5):519–27.
149. Chimanovitch I, et al. IgG1 and IgG3 are the major immunoglobulin subclasses targeting epitopes within the NC16A domain of BP180 in pemphigoid gestationis. J Invest Dermatol 1999;113(1):140–2.
150. Patton T, et al. IgG4 as the predominant IgG subclass in pemphigoides gestationis. J Cutan Pathol. 2006;33(4):299–302.
151. Tani N, Kimura Y, Koga H, Kawakami T, Ohata C, Ishii N, et al. Clinical and immunological profiles of 25 patients with pemphigoid gestationis. Br J Dermatol. 2015;172(1):120–9.
152. Roger D, Vaillant L, Fignon A, Pierre F, Bacq Y, Brechot J-F, et al. Specific pruritic diseases of pregnancy: a prospective study of 3192 pregnant women. Arch Dermatol. 1994;130(6):734–9.

153. Hallaji Z, Mortazavi H, Ashtari S, Nikoo A, Abdollahi M, Nasimi M. Pemphigoid gestationis: clinical and histologic features of twenty-three patients. Int J Womens Dermatol. 2016;3(2):86–90.
154. Castro LA, Lundell RB, Krause PK, Gibson LE. Clinical experience in pemphigoid gestationis: report of 10 cases. J Am Acad Dermatol. 2006;55(5):823–8.
155. Jenkins RE, Jones SA, Black MM. Conversion of pemphigoid gestationis to bullous pemphigoid--two refractory cases highlighting this association. Br J Dermatol. 1996;135(4):595–8.
156. Al-Mutairi N, Sharma AK, Zaki A, El-Adawy E, Al-Sheltawy M, Nour-Eldin O. Maternal and neonatal pemphigoid gestationis. Clin Exp Dermatol. 2004;29(2):202–4.
157. Semkova K, Black M. Pemphigoid gestationis: current insights into pathogenesis and treatment. Eur J Obstet Gynecol Reprod Biol. 2009;145(2):138–44.
158. Shornick JK, Black MM. Fetal risks in herpes gestationis. J Am Acad Dermatol. 1992;26(1):63–8.
159. Chi CC, Wang SH, Charles-Holmes R, Ambros-Rudolph C, Powell J, Jenkins R, et al. Pemphigoid gestationis: early onset and blister formation are associated with adverse pregnancy outcomes. Br J Dermatol. 2009;160(6):1222–8.
160. Shornick JK, Black MM. Secondary autoimmune diseases in herpes gestationis (pemphigoid gestationis). J Am Acad Dermatol. 1992;26(4):563–6.
161. Cobo MF, Santi CG, Maruta CW, Aoki V. Pemphigoid gestationis: clinical and laboratory evaluation. Clinics (Sao Paulo). 2009;64(11):1043–7.
162. Huilaja L, Surcel HM, Bloigu A, Tasanen K. Elevated serum levels of BP180 antibodies in the first trimester of pregnancy precede gestational pemphigoid and remain elevated for a long time after remission of the disease. Acta Derm Venereol. 2015;95(7):843–4.
163. Sitaru C, Dahnrich C, Probst C, Komorowski L, Blocker I, Schmidt E, et al. Enzyme-linked immunosorbent assay using multimers of the 16th non-collagenous domain of the BP180 antigen for sensitive and specific detection of pemphigoid autoantibodies. Exp Dermatol. 2007;16(9):770–7.
164. Lehrhoff S, Pomeranz MK. Specific dermatoses of pregnancy and their treatment. Dermatol Ther. 2013;26(4):274–84.
165. Sävervall C, Sand FL, Thomsen SF. Pemphigoid gestationis: current perspectives. Clin Cosmet Investig Dermatol. 2017;10:441–9.
166. Butler DC, Heller MM, Murase JE. Safety of dermatologic medications in pregnancy and lactation: part II. Lactation. J Am Acad Dermatol. 2014;70(3):417.e1–10; quiz 27.
167. Doiron P, Pratt M. Antepartum intravenous immunoglobulin therapy in refractory pemphigoid gestationis: case report and literature review. J Cutan Med Surg. 2010;14(4):189–92.
168. Gan DC, Welsh B, Webster M. Successful treatment of a severe persistent case of pemphigoid gestationis with antepartum and postpartum intravenous immunoglobulin followed by azathioprine. Australas J Dermatol. 2012;53(1):66–9.
169. Braunstein I, Werth V. Treatment of dermatologic connective tissue disease and autoimmune blistering disorders in pregnancy. Dermatol Ther. 2013;26(4):354–63.
170. Marker M, Derfler K, Monshi B, Rappersberger K. Successful immunoapheresis of bullous autoimmune diseases: pemphigus vulgaris and pemphigoid gestationis. J Ger Soc Dermatol: JDDG. 2011;9(1):27–31.
171. Van de Wiel A, Hart HC, Flinterman J, Kerckhaert JA, Du Boeuff JA, Imhof JW. Plasma exchange in herpes gestationis. Br Med J. 1980;281(6247):1041–2.
172. Özdemir Ö, Atalay CR, Asgarova V, Ilgin BU. A resistant case of pemphigus gestationis successfully treated with cyclosporine. Interv Med Appl Sci. 2016;8(1):20–2.
173. Hern S, Harman K, Bhogal BS, Black MM. A severe persistent case of pemphigoid gestationis treated with intravenous immunoglobulins and cyclosporin. Clin Exp Dermatol. 1998;23(4):185–8.
174. Huilaja L, Makikallio K, Hannula-Jouppi K, Vakeva L, Hook-Nikanne J, Tasanen K. Cyclosporine treatment in severe gestational pemphigoid. Acta Derm Venereol. 2015;95(5):593–5.

175. Hapa A, Gurpinar A, Akan T, Gokoz O. A resistant case of pemphigus gestationis successfully treated with intravenous immunoglobulin plus cyclosporine. Int J Dermatol. 2014;53(4):e269–71.
176. Castle SP, Mather-Mondrey M, Bennion S, David-Bajar K, Huff C. Chronic herpes gestationis and antiphospholipid antibody syndrome successfully treated with cyclophosphamide. J Am Acad Dermatol. 1996;34(2 Pt 2):333–6.
177. Loo WJ, Dean D, Wojnarowska F. A severe persistent case of recurrent pemphigoid gestationis successfully treated with minocycline and nicotinamide. Clin Exp Dermatol. 2001;26(8):726–7.
178. Amato L, Coronella G, Berti S, Gallerani I, Moretti S, Fabbri P. Successful treatment with doxycycline and nicotinamide of two cases of persistent pemphigoid gestationis. J Dermatolog Treat. 2002;13(3):143–6.
179. Werth VP, Fivenson D, Pandya AG, Chen D, Rico MJ, Albrecht J, et al. Multicenter randomized, double-blind, placebo-controlled, clinical trial of dapsone as a glucocorticoid-sparing agent in maintenance-phase pemphigus vulgaris. Arch Dermatol. 2008;144(1):25–32.
180. Cianchini G, Masini C, Lupi F, Corona R, De Pita O, Puddu P. Severe persistent pemphigoid gestationis: long-term remission with rituximab. Br J Dermatol. 2007;157(2):388–9.
181. Yang A, Uhlenhake E, Murrell DF. Pemphigoid gestationis and intravenous immunoglobulin therapy. Int J Womens Dermatol. 2018;4(3):166–9.
182. Almeida FT, Sarabando R, Pardal J, Brito C. Pemphigoid gestationis successfully treated with intravenous immunoglobulin. BMJ Case Rep. 2018;2018:bcr-2018.
183. Nguyen T, Alraqum E, Razzaque Ahmed A. Positive clinical outcome with IVIg as monotherapy in recurrent pemphigoid gestationis. Int Immunopharmacol. 2015;26(1):1–3.
184. Rodrigues Cdos S, Filipe P, Solana Mdel M, Soares de Almeida L, Cirne de Castro J, Gomes MM. Persistent herpes gestationis treated with high-dose intravenous immunoglobulin. Acta Derm Venereol. 2007;87(2):184–6.
185. Kreuter A, Harati A, Breuckmann F, Appelhans C, Altmeyer P. Intravenous immune globulin in the treatment of persistent pemphigoid gestationis. J Am Acad Dermatol. 2004;51(6):1027–8.
186. Roth MM. Atopic eruption of pregnancy: a new disease concept. J Eur Acad Dermatol Venereol. 2009;23(12):1466–7.

Part II
Pre-Existing Skin Disease in Pregnancy

Chapter 3
Psoriasis

Daisy Danielle Yan and Lisa Pappas-Taffer

Epidemiology

Introduction

Psoriasis is a chronic, immune-mediated skin condition with a multifactorial etiology. Skin lesion appearance can vary by psoriasis type. Plaque-type psoriasis is characterized by well-defined, erythematous plaques with micaceous scale. It can be localized with only a few plaques, or it can involve a large percentage of the body's surface area including scalp, nails, and genitalia. Psoriasis is a systemic inflammatory condition, sometimes affecting joints (psoriatic arthritis) and increasing the risk of adverse cardiovascular outcomes [1]. Up to 20–30% of psoriasis patients will have psoriatic arthritis, which often necessitates systemic therapy. The prevalence of psoriasis in the US may be as high as 4.6%, and it can manifest at any age; however, the majority (75%) of psoriasis presents before 40 years of age. Prevalence between genders is roughly equal, but females have a younger mean of onset (14.8 years) compared to males (17.3), suggesting a role for sex hormones [2].

Disease Activity of Psoriasis

During pregnancy, the majority of psoriasis stabilizes or improves. Forty-five psoriasis patients with >10% BSA were assessed prospectively at 10, 20, and 30 weeks of pregnancy and post-partum. Improvement in lesions was noted in approximately

D. D. Yan · L. Pappas-Taffer (✉)
Department of Dermatology, University of Pennsylvania, Philadelphia, PA, USA
e-mail: Daisy.Yan@Pennmedicine.upenn.edu; Lisa.Pappas-Taffer@pennmedicine.upenn.edu

K. H. Tyler (ed.), *Cutaneous Disorders of Pregnancy*,
https://doi.org/10.1007/978-3-030-49285-4_3

half of patients, with approximately 25% of patients remaining stable. Only roughly 25% of the pregnant patients had worsened psoriasis. Among those who improved, there was a significant improvement, with an 83.8% reduction in psoriasis lesions from week 10 to 30 [3]. However, post-partum flares are not uncommon (occurring in 40–90% of patients), and 30–40% of women note the onset of psoriatic arthritis in either the post-partum or peri-menopausal period [4]. One theory for this waning and waxing course during pregnancy is the hormone-driven modulation of the immune system. It has been hypothesized that progesterone can directly affect keratinocytes, which possess estrogen and progesterone receptors [5]. There is also a shift from Type 1 T helper cell (T_H1) to Type 2 T helper cell (T_H2) immunity to prevent fetal rejection during pregnancy, which is thought to explain improvement in autoimmune T_H1-mediated diseases, such as psoriasis.

Pustular psoriasis of pregnancy (PPP) is a subset of generalized pustular psoriasis that occurs during the third trimester of pregnancy. PPP was originally called impetigo herpetiformis (IH), but IH is a misnomer, as PPP is not caused by bacterial or viral infections. PPP is characterized by coalescent pustules, eventual desquamation, and systemic symptoms such as fever, delirium, and diarrhea. Mother and fetus are at risk of electrolyte imbalances and secondary sepsis in severe cases. PPP generally resolves upon parturition but can recur in subsequent pregnancies.

Pregnancy Outcomes in Psoriasis

There is a paucity of rigorous data about the impact of psoriasis on pregnancy outcomes. A systemic review of 9 observational studies reported spontaneous abortion, caesarean delivery, low birth weight, macrosomia, large-for-gestational age, or prematurity/low birthweight as adverse pregnancy outcomes. However, there was no consistent relationship across studies linking psoriasis and adverse pregnancy outcomes [6]. One reason for this could be a failure to stratify psoriasis by severity. In patients with mild to moderate psoriasis, 3 prospective cohort studies found no increased risk for adverse birth outcomes, spontaneous abortions, or fetal death [7–9]. In patients with moderate to severe psoriasis, there was an increased risk for low birth weight and spontaneous abortions [7, 10, 11]. Most recently, a cross-sectional population-based cohort study was performed in which data was collected prospectively from Denmark and Sweden [12]. 8097 births were identified in 6103 women with psoriasis and 753 with psoriatic arthritis. An increased incidence of gestational diabetes, gestational hypertension, eclampsia, and elective and emergent cesarean section was noted in patients with severe psoriatic disease. Hence, more severe disease burden appears to correlate with poorer pregnancy outcomes. For PPP, close monitoring and early treatment is paramount, as placental insufficiency, intrauterine growth restriction, and fetal demise have been observed [13].

Treatment

For patients with mild to moderate psoriasis who are planning pregnancy or who become pregnant, the author (LPT) provides patients reassurance that 75% of patients will have stable to improved disease and that no or scaled back therapy could be an option. However, for patients with severe disease, the risk of NOT treating the psoriasis (i.e. poor pregnancy outcomes) may outweigh those of medications, and often continuation of therapy is advised.

Treatment of psoriasis during pregnancy should be tailored to minimize adverse effects on both the mother and fetus. Consensus guidelines are helpful but not absolute given the rapid explosion of new medications to treat moderate to severe psoriasis in the last 10 years. However, an agreed upon therapeutic ladder includes starting with topical agents, then phototherapy, then systemic agents.

First line treatment includes emollients and low-to-moderate potency topical steroids [14]. Although topical steroids were previously categorized as Federal Drug Administration (FDA) pregnancy category C (Table 1.1), large studies have demonstrated safety with no evidence of increased risk for congenital abnormalities or pregnancy loss. Extensive use of high potency topical steroids should be avoided, however, given a possible association with low birth weight with excessive absorption [15]. Topical therapy is an effective strategy for treating limited disease, typically 5–10% BSA or less (Fig. 3.1).

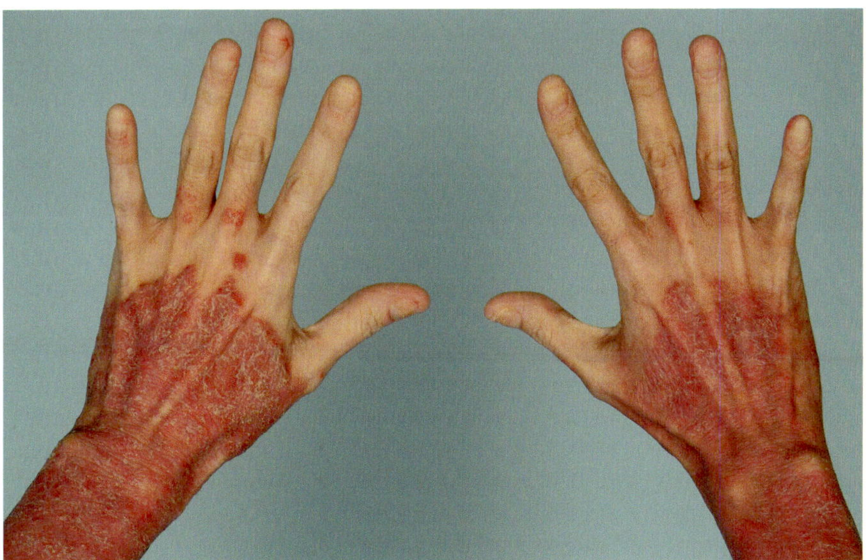

Fig. 3.1 Topical steroids are insufficient for widespread psoriasis (greater than 5–10% BSA). (Photo used with permission of Dr. Joel Gelfand, University of Pennsylvania)

Second line treatment is narrowband ultraviolet light phototherapy (nbUVB). Special precautions must be taken to avoid overheating and to supplement with folic acid, since high cumulative nbUVB doses can cause decreased levels of serum folate, theoretically increasing the risk of neural tube defects in the fetus [16]. Phototherapy is a great modality for those who prefer to avoid systemic therapy and can be continued after delivery to avoid post-partum disease flares.

Third line treatment includes cyclosporine (CSA) and anti-Tumor Necrosis Factor (TNF) agents. While cyclosporine has not been studied in the context of psoriasis and pregnancy, transplant literature has shown no association with congenital malformations, and it is overall safe [17]. However, an increased risk for maternal hypertension, low birth weight, and prematurity have been noted [14]. Cyclosporine may be favored in situations where short-term control is needed given its short half-life and rapid onset of effect.

Anti-TNFs, also considered third line treatment, are considered safe during pregnancy (previously FDA pregnancy category B). Prospective observational studies in both psoriasis and other inflammatory conditions demonstrate that exposure in the first trimester was not associated with an increased risk of teratogenicity. However, a recent systematic review in British Journal of Dermatology suggested a trend toward a drug-specific increase in the risk of congenital malformations and preterm births [18]. This review included 4 studies with 1300 women exposed to anti-TNFs 3 months prior to pregnancy. Three of the studies showed an increased risk of congenital malformations and preterm births. However, they did not control for co-therapies, the results did not meet statistical significance, and there was no specific constellation of malformations.

How does one maximize safety of a TNF-inhibitor? Via choice of agent and timepoint during pregnancy. Anti-TNF agents vary in composition, although most are composed of IgG1 antibodies. IgG1 antibodies can cross the placenta in varying amounts depending on the trimester. IgG1 antibodies (hence most anti-TNF agents) are actively transported by the neonatal fragment Fc receptor on the placenta, with IgG1 transferring better than other antibody subtypes. During the 1st trimester, there is no crossing of the placenta. During the 2nd trimester, transport begins as early as 13 weeks of gestation but significantly increases after 20 weeks, with IgG1 actively transported across the placenta by the 3rd trimester. This transportation delay makes congenital malformations unlikely (despite the recent study cited above), as fetal organogenesis occurs in the first trimester. However, one can further maximize anti-TNF agent safety during pregnancy via choice of specific anti-TNF agents, with those lacking the IgG portion being ideal. Hence, etanercept (a fusion protein of the TNF receptor) and certolizumab (a biologic that lacks the IgG Fc portion) are the anti-TNF agents of choice in pregnancy.

Newborn infants born to mothers treated with anti-TNF agents should be considered immunosuppressed due to placental passage. Reports have detected adalimumab at 11 weeks and infliximab at 7 months in infant blood after delivery [19]. An isolated case report of in utero infliximab exposure resulted in the death of a 3 month old due to vaccine-induced disseminated BCG infection [20]. Hence, the CDC recommends postponing live vaccines (e.g. rotavirus) until infants are ≥6 months of age. Non-live vaccinations are still effective and should be delivered without delays.

Regarding lactation, monoclonal antibodies used in biologic therapies have poor oral bioavailability due to their large molecular size. Therefore, gastrointestinal absorption is theoretically limited. In several studies, infliximab was undetectable in the breastmilk of nursing mothers or sera of their newborn children [21]. Hence, there is no contraindication to nursing while on an anti-TNF agent.

Due to PPP's potential for life-threatening complications, first line treatment is prompt initiation of systemic corticosteroids or cyclosporine [22]. For mild cases of PPP, adequate control can be achieved at corticosteroid dosages of <30 mg/day. For more severe cases, corticosteroid dosage can be increased to up to 60–80 mg/day. For PPP, cyclosporine dosage is 2–3 mg/kg body weight/day. Phototherapy, specifically nbUVB, can be helpful, but acts more often as an adjunctive therapy. Fetal monitoring and maternal electrolyte, calcium, vitamin D, and albumin levels should be followed closely.

Other Biologics

A new influx of biologics has joined the traditional arsenal of psoriasis treatments. These include anti-IL 12/23 agents (ustekinumab), anti-IL-17a agents (secukinumab, ixekizumab, brodalumab), and anti-IL-23 agents (guselkumab, tildrakizumab). All anti-TNFs, ustekinumab, and secukinumab were labelled as FDA pregnancy cateogory B. The remaining newer agents came to market following the discontinuation of FDA pregnancy categories. Based on preliminary data, there are no concerns for congenital malformations, and these newer biologics are thought to be safe in pregnancy based on animal studies and reports of pregnancy in patients already being treated with these agents. However, given the small number of reports, treatment during pregnancy should be considered on a case by case basis. In contrast, apremilast, the oral PDE-4 inhibitor, carries a previous FDA pregnancy category C due to an increased risk of miscarriage based on animal studies [23].

Considerations for Biologic Therapy [24, 25]

- Consensus: biologics appear safe, but there are ways to maximize safety
- Pre-pregnancy planning includes consideration of disease severity, timing of drug initiation and timing of drug termination
- Many recommend stopping once pregnancy confirmed
- Most recommend stopping by or at 30 weeks gestational age
- Consider agent: Certolizumab or Etanercept preferable

Therapeutics to Avoid

Certain therapeutics must be avoided during pregnancy. In addition to avoiding apremilast as a treatment for psoriasis during pregnancy, other agents routinely used to treat psoriasis are contraindicated in pregnancy. Furthermore, certain agents need to be avoided 1 month to 3 years prior to pregnancy, so discussing reproductive goals for all patients of reproductive age is important. Methotrexate must be stopped 3 months prior to pregnancy due to its folate-depleting effects. Acitretin must be stopped 3 years prior to pregnancy. Psoralen plus ultraviolet A light phototherapy (PUVA) was previously FDA pregnancy category C due to mutagenic potential and increased risk of low birth weight babies [26]. Topical medications to be avoided are tazarotene (previous FDA pregnancy category X), extensive application of salicylic acid (potential for salicylate toxicity), anthralin and coal tar (both contain carcinogenic polycyclic aromatic hydrocarbons), and extensive application of calcipotriene (risk for hypercalcemia with overuse). Safety studies of tacrolimus were based on oral consumption, and it was previously classified as FDA pregnancy category C. The topical form has less absorption than topical steroids and is generally considered safe, but various fields have discordant opinions on its safety; transplant and connective tissue disease literature find it similar to cyclosporine in safety, while some of the psoriasis literature does not recommend its use.

Psoriasis Summary

- Typically improves in pregnancy
- Baseline risk to pregnancy outcomes based on inflammatory burden
- Expect post-partum flares
- Treatment Ladder: Topicals > nbUVB > CSA or anti-TNFs
- Anti-TNFs
  - Etanercept or certolizumab safest
  - For those who want to get pregnant with mild/moderate disease – can stop once conceives
  - For severe disease, continue therapy until 30 weeks then stop (vs continue after discussion of risks and benefits)
  - Delay live vaccines for infant
- Avoid: apremilast, methotrexate, PUVA, tazarotene, anthralin, and coal tar; avoid extensive application of salicylic acid and calcipotriene

In terms of disease activity, psoriasis tends to stabilize or improve during pregnancy and flare post-partum. Moderate-to-severe psoriasis and PPP have potential for worse pregnancy outcomes; therefore, it is crucial to have thorough and timely pre-pregnancy counseling. A study conducted by Maccari et al. investigating the preconceptions of 152 French dermatologists and patients with psoriasis underscores the necessity of broaching this topic [27]. Only half of the dermatologists were aware that the highest risk period of pregnancy was the first trimester, one-third were up to date on current treatment guidelines, and only 7.89% reported making a joint treatment decision with a patient's obstetrician. Reproductive goals should be an ongoing discussion, and discussion of the risks and benefits of treatment as well as risks of non-treatment is critical. Communication with a patient's obstetrician is also paramount.

Generally, skin directed therapy is typically preferred. If initiating anti-TNF therapy for psoriasis, consider etanercept or certolizumab. Based on severity, continuation of a patient's current biologic is an option. Overall, published guidelines for treatment of psoriasis in pregnancy are useful but not absolute.

References

1. Husni ME. Comorbidities in psoriatic arthritis. Rheum Dis Clin. 2015;41(4):677–98.
2. Levi SS, Ramot Y. Gender differences in psoriasis. In: Tur E, Maibach HI, editors. Gender and dermatology. Cham: Springer International Publishing; 2018. p. 63–81.
3. Murase JE, Chan KK, Garite TJ, Cooper DM, Weinstein GD. Hormonal effect on psoriasis in pregnancy and post partum. Arch Dermatol. 2005;141(5):601–6.
4. Tauscher AE, Fleischer AB, Phelps KC, Feldman SR. Psoriasis and pregnancy. J Cutan Med Surg Inc Med Surg Dermatol. 2002;6(6):561–70.
5. Ruiz V, Manubens E, Puig L. Psoriasis in pregnancy: a review (I). Actas Dermosifiliogr (English Edition). 2014;105(8):734–43.
6. Bobotsis R, Gulliver W, Monaghan K, Lynde C, Fleming P. Psoriasis and adverse pregnancy outcomes: a systematic review of observational studies. Br J Dermatol. 2016;175(3):464–72.
7. Yang Y-W, Chen C-S, Chen Y-H, Lin H-C. Psoriasis and pregnancy outcomes: a nationwide population-based study. J Am Acad Dermatol. 2011;64(1):71–7.
8. Lima XT, Janakiraman V, Hughes MD, Kimball AB. The impact of psoriasis on pregnancy outcomes. J Investig Dermatol. 2012;132(1):85–91.
9. Harder E, Andersen A-MN, Kamper-Jørgensen M, Skov L. No increased risk of fetal death or prolonged time to pregnancy in women with psoriasis. J Invest Dermatol. 2014;134(6):1747.
10. Ben-David G, Sheiner E, Hallak M, Levy A. Pregnancy outcome in women with psoriasis. J Reprod Med. 2008;53(3):183–7.
11. Cohen-Barak E, Nachum Z, Rozenman D, Ziv M. Pregnancy outcomes in women with moderate-to-severe psoriasis. J Eur Acad Dermatol Venereol. 2011;25(9):1041–7.
12. Bröms G, Haerskjold A, Granath F, Kieler H, Pedersen L, Berglind IA. Effect of maternal psoriasis on pregnancy and birth outcomes: a population-based cohort study from Denmark and Sweden. Acta Derm Venereol. 2018;98(7–8):728–34.
13. Oumeish OY, Parish JL. Impetigo herpetiformis. Clin Dermatol. 2006;24(2):101–4.
14. Bae Y-SC, Van Voorhees AS, Hsu S, Korman NJ, Lebwohl MG, Young M, et al. Review of treatment options for psoriasis in pregnant or lactating women: from the Medical Board of the National Psoriasis Foundation. J Am Acad Dermatol. 2012;67(3):459–77.
15. Chi CC, Wang SH, Wojnarowska F, Kirtschig G, Davies E, Bennett C. Safety of topical corticosteroids in pregnancy. JAMA Dermatol. 2016;152(8):934–93.
16. El-Saie LT, Rabie AR, Kamel MI, Seddeik AK, Elsaie ML. Effect of narrowband ultraviolet B phototherapy on serum folic acid levels in patients with psoriasis. Lasers Med Sci. 2011;26(4):481–5.

17. Colla L, Diena D, Rossetti M, Manzione AM, Marozio L, Benedetto C, et al. Immunosuppression in pregnant women with renal disease: review of the latest evidence in the biologics era. J Nephrol. 2018;31(3):361–83.
18. Pottinger E, Woolf RT, Exton LS, Burden AD, Nelson-Piercy C, Smith CH. Exposure to biological therapies during conception and pregnancy: a systematic review. Br J Dermatol. 2018;178(1):95–102.
19. Julsgaard M, Christensen LA, Gibson PR, Gearry RB, Fallingborg J, Hvas CL, et al. Concentrations of adalimumab and infliximab in mothers and newborns, and effects on infection. Gastroenterology. 2016;151(1):110–9.
20. Cheent K, Nolan J, Shariq S, Kiho L, Pal A, Arnold J. Case report: fatal case of disseminated BCG infection in an infant born to a mother taking infliximab for Crohn's disease. J Crohn's Colitis. 2010;4(5):603–5.
21. Lund T, Thomsen SF. Use of TNF-inhibitors and ustekinumab for psoriasis during pregnancy: a patient series. Dermatol Ther. 2017;30(3):e12454.
22. Trivedi MK, Vaughn AR, Murase JE. Pustular psoriasis of pregnancy: current perspectives. Int J Women's Health. 2018;10:109.
23. Otezla (Apremilast) [package insert]. Summit: Celgene Pharmaceutical Companies; 2017.
24. Puig L, Barco D, Alomar A. Treatment of psoriasis with anti-TNF drugs during pregnancy: case report and review of the literature. Dermatology. 2010;220(1):71–6.
25. Mahadevan U, Wolf DC, Dubinsky M, Cortot A, Lee SD, Siegel CA, et al. Placental transfer of anti–tumor necrosis factor agents in pregnant patients with inflammatory bowel disease. Clin Gastroenterol Hepatol. 2013;11(3):286–92.
26. Murase JE, Heller MM, Butler DC. Safety of dermatologic medications in pregnancy and lactation: part I. Pregnancy. J Am Acad Dermatol. 2014;70(3):401.e1–e14.
27. Maccari F, Fougerousse AC, Esteve E, Frumholtz L, Parier J, Hurabielle C, et al. Crossed looks on the dermatologist's position and the patient's preoccupations as to psoriasis and pregnancy: preliminary results of the PREGNAN-PSO study. J Eur Acad Dermatol Venereol. 2019;33(5):880–5.

Chapter 4
Autoimmune Connective Tissue Diseases

Daisy Danielle Yan and Lisa Pappas-Taffer

Introduction

Autoimmune connective tissue diseases (CTDs) encompass a wide range of dermatological conditions such as cutaneous lupus, dermatomyositis, systemic sclerosis, and morphea. Although they fall under the same umbrella, the risk of flare during pregnancy differs among specific CTDs. There are no consensus guidelines for treating cutaneous CTDs in pregnancy. Recommended treatment algorithms are mainly based on expert opinion [1, 2].

Lupus Erythematosus

Epidemiology

Introduction

Cutaneous lupus erythematous (CLE) is an autoimmune skin condition with a multifactorial etiology. Skin lesion appearance can vary by CLE type. Discoid lupus erythematosus (DLE), the most common form of chronic cutaneous lupus (CCLE), is characterized by scaly, erythematous plaques and papules and that cause scarring and alopecia as sequelae (Fig. 4.1). Other CCLE subtypes, such as tumid lupus and lupus panniculitis, are less common. Subcutaneous lupus erythematosus (SCLE) lesions can have an annular or papulosquamous appearance but are generally photodistributed. Acute cutaneous lupus (ACLE) is characterized by malar erythema and

D. D. Yan · L. Pappas-Taffer (✉)
Department of Dermatology, University of Pennsylvania, Philadelphia, PA, USA
e-mail: Daisy.Yan@Pennmedicine.upenn.edu; Lisa.Pappas-Taffer@pennmedicine.upenn.edu

K. H. Tyler (ed.), *Cutaneous Disorders of Pregnancy*,
https://doi.org/10.1007/978-3-030-49285-4_4

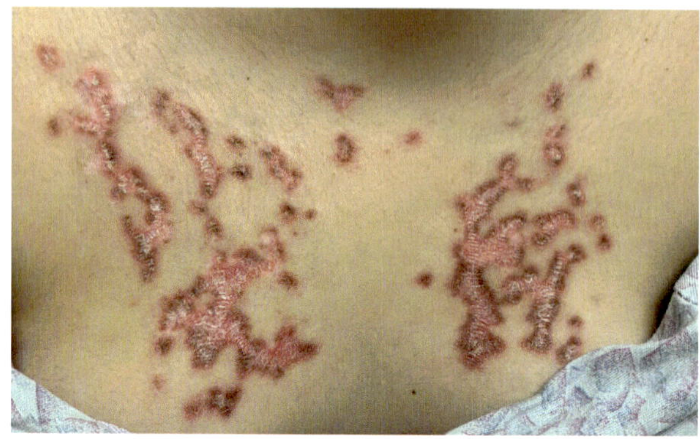

Fig. 4.1 Discoid lupus of the chest. Photo used with permission of Dr. Victoria Werth, University of Pennsylvania

only occurs in the setting of systemic lupus erythematosus (SLE) flares. In contrast to ACLE, all other CLE subtypes can occur in the setting of SLE or as isolated skin disease in the absence of SLE. Various studies have reported that approximately 20% to 25% of newly diagnosed CLE patients will eventually progress to SLE [3]. Hence, 75–80% of CLE patients will never develop SLE but should be routinely screened. In general, CLE is equally as prevalent as SLE, with incidence rates ranging from 1.43 to 4.30 per 100,000 [4, 5]. Females are disproportionately affected by lupus, with a ratio of 6:1 for SLE and 3:1 for CLE when compared to men. The age of onset is primarily during the reproductive years, which makes treatment more salient. Fortunately, lupus in pregnancy is well-studied with regard to SLE, and we can extrapolate much of what we know about SLE for CLE.

Disease Activity of Lupus in Pregnancy

Literature regarding whether SLE worsens during pregnancy is contradictory, but it is often quoted that 50% of SLE patients will experience a flare during pregnancy [6, 7]. Most flares are not severe and typically manifest similarly to pre-pregnancy flares [8, 9]. While flares can occur anytime, the third trimester and the post-partum period are higher risk. Risk depends on disease activity 6 to 12 months pre-conception [10, 11].

Pregnancy Outcomes in Lupus

Compared to a healthy population, SLE patients are at higher risk for preeclampsia, thrombosis, preterm delivery, fetal growth restriction, and fetal loss [12, 13]. In one study which aimed to identify risk factors for adverse pregnancy outcomes in SLE, 385 multi-ethnic and multi-racial pregnant females with inactive or stable mild to moderate SLE were followed prospectively during pregnancy in 8 clinical centers across the US and Canada [14]. It showed that <5% had severe flares in the second or third trimesters, and the probability of a negative pregnancy outcome was <8%

for women without risk factors during the first trimester. Risk factors for adverse pregnancy outcomes included baseline hypertension, positive lupus anti-coagulant, active SLE, flares in the second or third trimester, and non-white ethnic origin. Women of non-white origin had more than double the risk of developing one or more adverse pregnancy outcomes; women of African (N = 78) and Hispanic (N = 58) descent had poor fetal outcomes in 27.4% and 20.6% of their pregnancies, respectively. Serologic data such as complements and anti-dsDNA did not correlate with poor outcomes. This study was quite reassuring in that it showed that inactive or stable mild to moderate SLE patients only rarely experience severe disease flares and overall have favorable pregnancy outcomes. It is unclear why women of non-white origin had a higher risk for adverse pregnancy outcomes, so this topic warrants further research.

Although SLE in pregnancy has been well studied, there are fewer studies evaluating pregnancy outcomes for those with isolated cutaneous disease. There are currently only two studies in the literature addressing cutaneous lupus erythematosus (CLE) and pregnancy outcomes. Both demonstrated that pregnancy outcomes in CLE were more favorable than SLE. The first study, a 2 center prospective cohort comparative study of CLE (n = 67), SLE (n = 67), and controls (n = 67), found similar pregnancy outcomes in CLE patients when compared to healthy controls [15]. In the second study, SLE patients who only had mucocutaneous involvement, such as malar rash, oral/nasal ulcers, and photosensitivity, had similar pregnancy outcomes to healthy controls [12].

Treatment

Treatment of CLE

Counselling and ongoing discussion of reproductive goals is crucial with all CLE patients of childbearing age. Understanding their goals can help in choosing appropriate treatment modalities and ensuring optimal disease control for at least 6 months prior to conception. While SLE patients should be classified as high risk obstetric patients, CLE patients with no systemic involvement should not [16]. The status of anti-SSA/SSB and antiphospholipid antibodies should be established given risk for neonatal lupus and increased risk for maternal and fetal morbidity, respectively.

The first line of treatment for CLE is photoprotection and skin-directed therapy [1]. Low to medium potency topical steroids and calcineurin inhibitors are recommended, while potent topical and intralesional steroids should be used sparingly. Calcineurin inhibitors have less absorption than topical steroids. Second line treatment is hydroxychloroquine (HCQ), which has been shown to reduce the risk of neonatal lupus, prematurity, and intrauterine growth restriction (IUGR) in SLE. HCQ is continued pre-pregnancy when topical therapy is insufficient, systemic manifestations are present, or the patient has a history of positive anti-SSA/SSB antibodies [17, 18]. Of note, there are no reports of fetal ocular toxicity with intrauterine HCQ exposure [19]. The third line treatment is azathioprine, which is added if HCQ is insufficient. Azathioprine can be continued if started pre-pregnancy, and it is the agent of choice if switching from contraindicated oral agents. Classically, azathioprine was previously labeled Federal Drug Administration (FDA) pregnancy category D (Table 1.1), but data from the transplant population is reassuring [20]. There is no evidence of congenital malformations, spontaneous abortions, or stillbirths, but the reported case numbers may not be sufficient. Recently, azathioprine exposure was suggested to impose a slightly increased risk of atrial or ventricular septal defects in the fetus [21]. Fourth line treatment is intravenous immunoglobulin (IVIG).

Therapies to avoid in pregnancy include chloroquine, methotrexate, mycophenolate mofetil, cyclophosphamide, and acitretin [2]. Chloroquine has a higher placental drug concentration than HCQ, although a Cochrane meta-analysis supports chloroquine safety in the setting of malaria prophylaxis at lower doses [22]. Methotrexate is an abortifacient, has teratogenic properties, and is a previous FDA pregnancy category X. Methotrexate needs to be discontinued 3 months prior to conception. Mycophenolate mofetil is a previous FDA pregnancy category D drug that is teratogenic, and it needs to be discontinued 6 weeks before conception. Cyclophosphamide is former FDA pregnancy category D and can cause miscarriages [23]. Acitretin, previously FDA pregnancy category X, needs to be discontinued 3 years prior to conception.

Dermatomyositis

Epidemiology

Introduction

Dermatomyositis (DM) is a multisystem autoimmune condition that classically involves inflammation of the skin and muscle but can also affect the lungs. Skin findings consist of symmetric pink to violaceous patches or plaques and poikiloderma (hypopigmented, hyperpigmented, and erythematous mottling) on the extensor surfaces, pink papules overlying the joints of the fingers (Atrophic papules of DM, also referred to as Gottron's papules) (Fig. 4.2), and a violacous rash of the eyelids (heliotrope rash). Severe cases can present as erythrodermic (confluent red rash of the entire body) or ulcerated. Proximal muscle weakness with elevated serum creatinine phosphokinase (CPK) and aldolase is often seen, but there are amyopathic and hypomyopathic DM subtypes without muscle involvement. While the etiology is still unknown, internal malignancies and other factors such as pregnancy, drugs or supplements, and infectious agents have been reported as triggers. Lung disease is usually of the interstitial lung disease (ILD) variety. The incidence

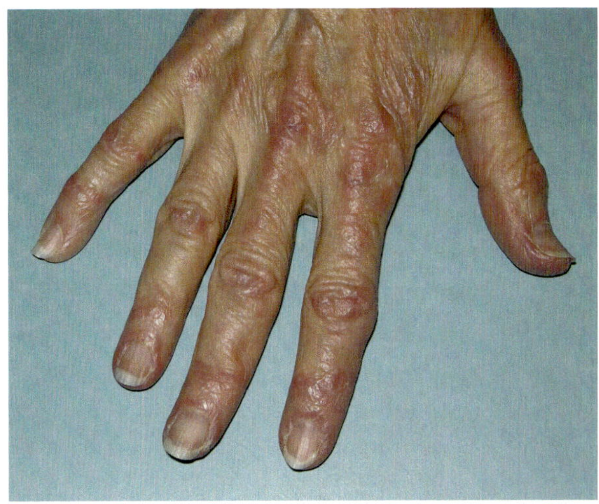

Fig. 4.2 Gottron's papules, characterized by erythema along the bony prominences, are a pathognomonic sign of dermatomyositis. Photo used with permission of Dr. Victoria Werth, University of Pennsylvania

of dermatomyositis is rising, although it has previously been reported as 10 per one million [24]. Similar to lupus, DM disproportionately affects females over males. Age of onset is usually bimodal, with both juvenile and adult types; the adult age of onset is usually early 50's [25].

Disease Activity of Dermatomyositis in Pregnancy

Literature regarding DM during pregnancy is scarce, since only 10–15% of DM cases occur during the reproductive years. Although data mostly consists of case reports and smaller studies, they suggest that DM stabilizes or improves during pregnancy and flares postpartum [26, 27]. A study from Brazil of 9 pregnant patients with DM found only 1 flare amongst 13 total documented pregnancies [26]. Another collaborative study from University of Pennsylvania and Stanford observed 10 DM patients over 23 pregnancies, and disease activity improved during pregnancy among all but one [27]. However, a recent case series found an association with pregnancy-induced dermatomyositis and TIF1-gamma antibody positivity [28].

Pregnancy Outcomes in Dermatomyositis

Adverse pregnancy outcomes in DM include IUGR, prematurity, and fetal loss, but there is minimal risk to the fetus if DM is well-controlled pre-conception. Worsened fetal prognosis is associated with severe maternal disease, flares during pregnancy, and first onset of disease during pregnancy [26, 29, 30].

Treatment

Treatment of Dermatomyositis in Pregnancy

Therapies for DM during pregnancy are similar to CLE, but muscle and lung involvement must be taken into account [1]. Photoprotection is recommended regardless of disease severity. For mild skin-limited disease, low to medium potency topical steroids and/or topical calcineurin inhibitors are first line. For recalcitrant skin disease, HCQ can be added. For muscle and/or lung involvement or skin involvement refractory to HCQ, either oral corticosteroids or IVIG can be added [31, 32]. Oral steroids must be dosed at the lowest effective dose for rapid control, and azathioprine can be added to keep the maintenance steroid dose at less than 20 mg of prednisone per day. IVIG is dosed at 1 to 2 grams per kilogram (g/kg) divided over 2 to 5 consecutive days monthly. If the treating physician anticipates that a patient's DM might require an extended course of corticosteroids, IVIG would be the preferred agent.

Summary

In terms of disease activity, dermatomyositis tends to stabilize or improve during pregnancy and flare post-partum. CLE can flare, but pre-conception disease control reduces risks in pregnancy. For pregnancy outcomes in CTDs, higher risks for fetal mortality mirrors disease activity; therefore, it is crucial to have thorough and timely pre-pregnancy counseling. Reproductive goals should be an ongoing discussion, and a discussion of the risks and benefits of treatment as well as risks of non-treatment is critical. Communication with a patient's obstetrician is essential.

Before starting treatment, optimizing comorbidities and ensuring 6 months of controlled disease activity prior to conception will minimize potential risks during pregnancy. It is also important to know the patient's anti-SSA/SSB and antiphospholipid status in CTD to stratify pregnancy risk and treatment choice. Generally, skin-directed therapy is preferred. In CTD, systemic concerns warrant continuation of HCQ or azathioprine, which are shown to improve fetal outcomes. Overall, published guidelines for autoimmune CTD are useful but not absolute.

References

1. Braunstein I, Werth V. Treatment of dermatologic connective tissue disease and autoimmune blistering disorders in pregnancy. Dermatol Ther. 2013;26(4):354–63.
2. Wan J, Imadojemu S, Werth VP. Management of rheumatic and autoimmune blistering disease in pregnancy and postpartum. Clin Dermatol. 2016;34(3):344–52.
3. Wieczorek IT, Propert KJ, Okawa J, Werth VP. Systemic symptoms in the progression of cutaneous to systemic lupus erythematosus. JAMA Dermatol. 2014;150(3):291–6.

4. Baek YS, Park SH, Baek J, Roh JY, Kim HJ. Cutaneous lupus erythematosus and its association with systemic lupus erythematosus: a nationwide population-based cohort study in Korea. J Dermatol. 2019.
5. Petersen MP, Möller S, Bygum A, Voss A, Bliddal M. Epidemiology of cutaneous lupus erythematosus and the associated risk of systemic lupus erythematosus: a nationwide cohort study in Denmark. Lupus. 2018;27(9):1424–30.
6. Chen JS, Roberts CL, Simpson JM, March LM. Pregnancy outcomes in women with rare autoimmune diseases. Arthrit Rheumatol. 2015;67(12):3314–23.
7. Ruiz-Irastorza G, Khamashta MA, Castellino G, Hughes GR. Systemic lupus erythematosus. Lancet. 2001;357(9261):1027–32.
8. Tedeschi SK, Massarotti E, Guan H, Fine A, Bermas BL, Costenbader KH. Specific systemic lupus erythematosus disease manifestations in the six months prior to conception are associated with similar disease manifestations during pregnancy. Lupus. 2015;24(12):1283–92.
9. Borella E, Lojacono A, Gatto M, Andreoli L, Taglietti M, Iaccarino L, et al. Predictors of maternal and fetal complications in SLE patients: a prospective study. Immunol Res. 2014;60(2–3):170–6.
10. Singh AG, Chowdhary VR. Pregnancy-related issues in women with systemic lupus erythematosus. Int J Rheum Dis. 2015;18(2):172–81.
11. Aggarwal N, Raveendran A, Suri V, Chopra S, Sikka P, Sharma A. Pregnancy outcome in systemic lupus erythematosus: Asia's largest single Centre study. Arch Gynecol Obstet. 2011;284(2):281–5.
12. Ateka-Barrutia O, Khamashta M. The challenge of pregnancy for patients with SLE. Lupus. 2013;22(12):1295–308.
13. Østensen M, Andreoli L, Brucato A, Cetin I, Chambers C, Clowse ME, et al. State of the art: reproduction and pregnancy in rheumatic diseases. Autoimmun Rev. 2015;14(5):376–86.
14. Buyon JP, Kim MY, Guerra MM, Laskin CA, Petri M, Lockshin MD, et al. Predictors of pregnancy outcomes in patients with lupus: a cohort study. Ann Intern Med. 2015;163(3):153–63.
15. Hamed HO, Ahmed SR, Alzolibani A, Kamal MM, Mostafa MS, Gamal RM, et al. Does cutaneous lupus erythematosus have more favorable pregnancy outcomes than systemic disease? A two-center study. Acta Obstet Gynecol Scand. 2013;92(8):934–42.
16. Lateef A, Petri M. Managing lupus patients during pregnancy. Best Pract Res Clin Rheumatol. 2013;27(3):435–47.
17. Salinas MÁS, Cruz AB, Castañeda ARC, Quezada LJJ, Arce-Salinas CA, Nemegyei JÁ, et al. Clinical practice guidelines for the management of pregnancy in women with autoimmune rheumatic diseases of the Mexican College of Rheumatology. Part II. Reumatología Clínica (English Edition). 2015;11(5):305–15.
18. Leroux M, Desveaux C, Parcevaux M, Julliac B, Gouyon J-B, Dallay D, et al. Impact of hydroxychloroquine on preterm delivery and intrauterine growth restriction in pregnant women with systemic lupus erythematosus: a descriptive cohort study. Lupus. 2015;24(13):1384–91.
19. Tincani A, Rebaioli CB, Frassi M, Taglietti M, Gorla R, Cavazzana I, et al. Pregnancy and autoimmunity: maternal treatment and maternal disease influence on pregnancy outcome. Autoimmun Rev. 2005;4(7):423–8.
20. Murase JE, Heller MM, Butler DC. Safety of dermatologic medications in pregnancy and lactation: Part I. Pregnancy. Journal of the American Academy of Dermatology. 2014;70(3):401. e1–e14.
21. Natekar A, Pupco A, Bozzo P, Koren G. Safety of azathioprine use during pregnancy.
22. Radeva-Petrova D, Kayentao K, ter Kuile FO, Sinclair D, Garner P. Drugs for preventing malaria in pregnant women in endemic areas: any drug regimen versus placebo or no treatment. Cochrane Database Syst Rev. 2014.
23. Clowse ME, Magder L, Petri M. Cyclophosphamide for lupus during pregnancy. Lupus. 2005;14(8):593–7.
24. Bendewald MJ, Wetter DA, Li X, Davis MD. Incidence of dermatomyositis and clinically amyopathic dermatomyositis: a population-based study in Olmsted County. Minnesota Archives Dermatol. 2010;146(1):26–30.

25. Gerami P, Schope JM, McDonald L, Walling HW, Sontheimer RD. A systematic review of adult-onset clinically amyopathic dermatomyositis (dermatomyositis sine myositis): a missing link within the spectrum of the idiopathic inflammatory myopathies. J Am Acad Dermatol. 2006;54(4):597–613.
26. Missumi LS, Souza FHCD, Andrade JQ, Shinjo SK. Pregnancy outcomes in dermatomyositis and polymyositis patients. Rev Bras Reumatol. 2015;55(2):95–102.
27. Miller G. In: Moore E, Valenzuela A, Chung L, Werth V, editors. Dermatomyositis and pregnancy: assessment of disease activity and pregnancy outcomes complicated by maternal Dermatomyositis: ACR/ARP Annual Meeting; 2016.
28. Oya K, Inoue S, Saito A, Nakamura Y, Ishitsuka Y, Fujisawa Y, et al. Pregnancy triggers the onset of anti-transcriptional intermediary factor 1γ antibody-positive dermatomyositis: a case series. Rheumatology. 2019.
29. Váncsa A, Ponyi A, Constantin T, Zeher M, Dankó K. Pregnancy outcome in idiopathic inflammatory myopathy. Rheumatol Int. 2007;27(5):435–9.
30. Chopra S, Suri V, Bagga R, Thami MR, Sharma A, Bambery P. Autoimmune inflammatory myopathy in pregnancy. Medscape J Med. 2008;10(1):17.
31. Linardaki G, Cherouvim E, Goni G, Boki KA. Intravenous immunoglobulin treatment for pregnancy-associated dermatomyositis. Rheumatol Int. 2011;31(1):113–5.
32. Mosca M, Strigini F, Carmignani A, D'ascanio A, Genazzani A, Bombardieri S. Pregnant patient with dermatomyositis successfully treated with intravenous immunoglobulin therapy. Arthritis Care Res. 2005;53(1):119–21.

Chapter 5
Atopic Dermatitis in Pregnancy

Blake Friedman and Lionel Bercovitch

Epidemiology

Atopic dermatitis is the most common skin condition in pregnancy, accounting for approximately 50% of all pregnant patients presenting with skin concerns [1, 2]. Approximately 27% of those diagnosed with atopic dermatitis of pregnancy carry a personal history of atopy or infantile atopic dermatitis, 50% report a family history of atopy, and 19% have children diagnosed with infantile atopic dermatitis [2]. However, recent studies suggest that up to 80% of those diagnosed with atopic dermatitis during pregnancy represent new diagnoses, with atopic dermatitis presenting for the first time in pregnancy [1, 2]. Of those who carry an existing diagnosis of atopic dermatitis, studies suggest disease exacerbations will occur in 52% to 61% of patients [3, 4]. The majority of these patients demonstrate deterioration in the second or third trimesters [5]. It should be noted that a small subset of patients with pre-existing atopic dermatitis demonstrate improvement of atopic dermatitis during pregnancy, with a recent small study reporting improvement in 4% of patients [3].

B. Friedman
Department of Dermatology, Warren Alpert Medical School of Brown University, Providence, RI, USA
e-mail: blake_friedman@brown.edu

L. Bercovitch (✉)
Department of Dermatology, Warren Alpert Medical School of Brown University, Providence, RI, USA

Division of Pediatric Dermatology, Hasbro Children's Hospital, Providence, RI, USA

Department of Medicine, Women and Infannts Hospital, Providence, RI, USA
e-mail: lionel_berccovitch@brown.edu

K. H. Tyler (ed.), *Cutaneous Disorders of Pregnancy*,
https://doi.org/10.1007/978-3-030-49285-4_5

Clinical Presentation

Atopic dermatitis of pregnancy classically presents with lesions in a "classical" atopic distribution, including the face, neck, décolleté, and flexural surfaces of the upper and lower extremities [1]. However, involvement of the trunk, hands and feet is relatively common [1]. Less frequently, patients may present with nipple, areolar, follicular or nummular eczema [1, 2]. Lesions can range from classic xerotic plaques to rarer presentations such as folliculocentric papules and sterile pustules [6]. Worsening of features associated with atopic dermatitis, including keratosis pilaris, xerosis and lichenification, occurs with increased frequency, especially in those with pre-existing atopic dermatitis [7].

Diagnosis

Atopic dermatitis of pregnancy is a clinical diagnosis. The diagnosis should be considered in the patient with a personal or family history of atopy with pruritic lesions in a classic atopic dermatitis distribution, as noted above. However, as previously noted, many patients lack a personal or family history of atopy, and atypical presentations of atopic dermatitis have been reported. Histopathologic findings are non-specific and are dependent on the stage and type of lesion biopsied [7]. Common histopathologic features reported include epidermal spongiosis, hyperkeratosis and parakeratosis, and a mononuclear perivascular infiltrate. Direct and indirect Immunofluorescence studies are negative [2]. Indeed, the diagnosis is usually made on clinical rather than histopathological grounds. Laboratory tests are non-definitive and not specific. While a subset of patients demonstrate elevation in serum immunoglobulin E (IgE) levels, the use of IgE as a diagnostic marker in pregnancy has been challenged due to a dearth of information regarding IgE regulation in pregnancy [1, 7]. A number of diagnostic criteria have been utilized in clinical studies, including Hanifin and Rajka's and U.K. Working party criteria. All diagnostic criteria were validated in hospital settings, populations settings, or both [7].

Pathogenesis

The pathogenesis of atopic dermatitis in pregnancy is likely multifactorial, involving immunologic, psychologic and iatrogenic factors. In pregnancy, the body must accommodate the developing fetus, antigenically different tissue, while maintaining immunocompetence against pathogens [8, 9]. Cytokines produced by the Type 1 T helper cell (Th1) subset, including interferon (IFN)-gamma and tumor necrosis factor (TNF)-alpha, inhibit trophoblast outgrowth as well as embryonic and fetal development [10]. In contrast, cytokines produced by the Type 2 T helper cell (Th2) subset, including Interleukin (IL)4, IL10, and IL13, are important for allograft tolerance, allowing for pregnancy maintenance and inhibiting a potentially deleterious Th1 response [11]. Thus, a switch from cell-mediated to humoral-mediated mechanism (Th1 to Th2 shift) during gestation plays a key role in placental immune tolerance [6]. As a result of this important immunologic shift in pregnancy, skin diseases that are that are Th2-mediated often worsen, whereas skin diseases that are Th1-mediated often improve during gestation [6]. It is widely accepted that atopic dermatitis is a Th2 dominant disease. Therefore, the shift towards a Th2 cytokine predominant state is thought to, at least in part, explain the increased severity and incidence of atopic dermatitis during pregnancy [6]. It should be noted that the immune response underlying atopic dermatitis is complicated, with Th1, Th17 and Th22 cells as well as numerous additional cytokines (i.e. IL25, IL31, and IL33) also implicated [12]. It is unclear if alterations in expression of these cytokines play a role in the worsening of atopic dermatitis during pregnancy [13].

In addition to immunologic changes, the pregnant mother is also exposed to emotional and physiologic stressors that may exacerbate pre-existing atopic dermatitis [14]. Atopic dermatitis is a complex condition with a known psychologic component, with stress and sleep deprivation contributing to (as well as being caused by) disease exacerbations [13]. Therefore, the stress and sleep pattern disruption associated with pregnancy may in part account of the worsening of atopic dermatitis in pregnancy.

The tendency to minimize medical interventions in pregnant patients may also play a role in the worsening of atopic dermatitis in pregnancy. While formal data on treatment patterns in pregnancy are lacking, providers and patients often reduce both topical and systemic interventions in pregnancy to minimize presumed risk to the fetus [13]. A recent Danish study demonstrated decreased use of both topical and systemic dermatologic interventions for atopic dermatitis during pregnancy as compared to prior to pregnancy. Of note, the reason for this reduction in interventions could not be elucidated from the collected data; thus, it is possible that the minimization of interventions could have been secondary to improvement or resolution of atopic dermatitis. However, within the studied cohort, there was increased use of prednisolone during pregnancy, which, the authors concluded, could indicate undertreatment of atopic dermatitis leading to need for rescue therapy with systemic treatments [15].

Importance

Given concern that treatment of atopic dermatitis could adversely affect the unborn fetus, it is not only important to closely evaluate the safety profile of available interventions but also consider the benefits of medical interventions to the mother and fetus. In addition to the clear improvement in comfort for the pregnant patient, treatment of atopic dermatitis in pregnancy may prevent deleterious outcomes for both the mother and fetus. Untreated atopic dermatitis puts the pregnant patient at risk of contracting secondary infections, including eczema herpeticum and *Staphylococcus aureus* infections. These infections are associated with morbidity to the pregnant patient and her unborn child, with maternal herpes simplex virus infection linked to premature delivery, miscarriage and intrauterine growth restriction [16]. Thus, while prompt treatment of these infections is warranted, prevention of such complications via adequate control of atopic dermatitis is beneficial. Additionally, there is a rare association between maternal atopic dermatitis and neonatal sepsis, a devastating condition with high mortality [15]. Further, a recent study demonstrated a significant association between antenatal atopy and the development of attention deficit hyperactive disorder-like symptoms in children [17]. Of note, an additional study showed a correlation between antenatal IL4 levels, known to be elevated in atopic dermatitis, and risk of attention deficit disorder in children; however, an independent relationship between antenatal atopic dermatitis and development of attention deficit disorder in children was not seen [18]. Thus, additional rigorous studies evaluating this relationship are needed. Moreover, deterioration of atopic dermatitis during pregnancy likely worsens maternal quality of life and anxiety. Interestingly, recent studies reported an association between maternal stress levels during pregnancy and atopic dermatitis in offspring [19, 20]. Studies examining the psychological effects of atopic dermatitis indicate significant improvement in psychologic distress with atopic dermatitis treatment [21]. Therefore, it is possible that through ameliorating stress associated with atopic dermatitis flares, effective treatment of maternal atopic dermatitis may indirectly decrease the risk of atopic dermatitis development in offspring. However, studies examining the incidence of atopic dermatitis in offspring born to mothers with adequately versus poorly controlled atopic dermatitis are lacking.

Treatment

Basic

In all patients with atopic disease, including pregnant individuals, routine management with emollients and use of mild cleansers is encouraged [22]. There is no evidence in the literature to support the use of any one emollient type; however, use of an emollient with high lipid content is recommended [13]. All emollients, including those containing urea (3–10%) and antipruritic agents (i.e. menthol and polidocanol), are deemed safe in pregnancy [23]. Patients should be instructed to proceed with lukewarm baths for hydration coupled with subsequent application of an occlusive emollient after patting the skin dry, which may decrease the necessity for additional treatments [24, 25]. Adequate cutaneous hydration facilitates transepidermal penetration of topical corticosteroids should additional therapies be required [5].

Topical Corticosteroids

Topical corticosteroids represent first line therapy for atopic dermatitis and are considered safe to use in pregnancy. They are categorized as a previous category C drug by the Food and Drug Administration (FDA) (Table 1.1) and considered safer than systemic corticosteroids given the low systemic absorption relative to systemic steroids [5]. While an earlier study demonstrated a significant association between topical corticosteroid use in pregnancy and orofacial clefting in infants born to exposed mothers, multiple large case-control studies failed to demonstrate any increased risk of this birth defect [26–28]. Additionally, studies examining the risk of preterm delivery failed to demonstrate increased risk in infants born to mothers with prenatal topical corticosteroid exposure; notably, these studies did note an inverse dose-dependent relationship between topical corticosteroids use and birth weight [29, 30]. A recent Cochrane review on the safety of topical corticosteroids in pregnancy noted a non-significant association between potent or very potent topical corticosteroid use and fetal low birth weight, but the studies evaluated were noted to be low-quality evidence [31]. Evidence-based guidelines for topical steroid use during pregnancy recommend use of low to medium potency topical steroids if effective, with high potency topical steroids used only for brief time periods. Of note, fluticasone propionate should be avoided in the pregnant patient, as it is the only topical corticosteroid of record not metabolized by the placenta [32]. Further, guidelines recommend against use of corticosteroids on areas with thinner skin and, consequently, greater rates of cutaneous absorption [32]. Should use of topical corticosteroids exceed 200 grams per month, additional treatments, such as phototherapy, should be considered [13]. Topical corticosteroids are generally considered safe in the breastfeeding mother. However, cleaning of the nipples immediately prior to breastfeeding is recommended [13].

Phototherapy

When atopic dermatitis is not responsive to emollients and topical low dose topical corticosteroids, providers should consider referral for phototherapy, with best results obtained using UVA (340–400 nm), broadband UV (UVA & UVB 290–400 nm), or narrow-band UVB (311 nm) [33, 34]. During UVA therapy in pregnancy, psoralens should be avoided due to concerns for teratogenicity [5]. While UV phototherapy is thought to be safe in pregnancy given relatively superficial penetration of UV rays, high cumulative doses of UVB (narrowband and broadband) has been associated with decreased folic acid, potentially increasing the risk of fetal neural tube defects, so folic acid supplementation is recommended [35, 36].

Topical Antibiotics

For localized superficial skin infections, topical mupirocin is safe to use in the pregnant patient. Systemic absorption of mupirocin is low, and no reports of harmful effects secondary to use in pregnancy exist in the literature [13]. However, it is not recommended for furunculosis or cellulitis or widespread impetiginization. Furthermore, muprocin resistance is becoming more prevalent worldwide.

Topical Calcineurin Inhibitors

The FDA categorizes calcineurin inhibitors as a previous pregnancy category C [5]. Unfortunately, rigorous studies on topical calcineurin inhibitor use in pregnancy are lacking. As such, our understanding of tacrolimus safety in pregnancy is largely derived from studies on systemic tacrolimus use in transplant patients. These studies suggest a possible association between systemic tacrolimus and fetal anomalies, prematurity and low birth weight; however, these results are likely confounded by the complicated health statuses of the transplant patient population in these studies [5, 37, 38]. Despite the above-noted association, topical tacrolimus is thought to be relatively safe due to low systemic absorption and may be used with caution on localized areas not responsive to more thoroughly investigated treatments, such as topical corticosteroids or phototherapy [39]. Of note, topical calcineurin inhibitors may be appropriate for use in the nursing mother due to low overall exposure to the infant; however, the nipple should be spared [40].

Systemic Steroids

The FDA classified systemic corticosteroids as former pregnancy category C [5]. Short courses of systemic corticosteroids may be considered for severe or recalcitrant atopic dermatitis in the third trimester when topical treatments have failed [22]. Systemic corticosteroids often produce dramatic improvement in symptoms; however, disease course may be complicated by severe rebound flare upon cessation of corticosteroid therapy [5]. When systemic corticosteroid treatment is deemed appropriate, non-halogenated corticosteroids such as prednisone, prednisolone and cortisol are preferred, as they are enzymatically inactivated in the placenta; in contrast, halogenated corticosteroids such as betamethasone and dexamethasone are not [23]. Due to this enzymatic inactivation, non-halogenated corticosteroids (prednisone and prednisolone) result in a favorable maternal-fetal gradient of approximately 10:1 [41]. Given low fetal exposure, the risk of fetal and neonatal adrenal suppression is thought to be low [41].

Numerous studies have examined the effect of in-utero corticosteroid exposure on the developing fetus, with variable results. A large retrospective study exploring the effect of *in utero* exposure to numerous courses of corticosteroids suggested a possible link to preterm birth and gastroesophageal reflux [42]. Additional studies noted a possible association between repetitive corticosteroid use in pregnancy, low birth weight, and intrauterine growth restriction [43, 44]. A single study noted an increased risk of cerebral palsy with repetitive versus single corticosteroid course exposure [44]. However, another two-year follow up study examining the same question failed to demonstrate any association between repetitive courses of corticosteroids and major disability, body size, blood pressure, health services utilization, or respiratory morbidity. Of note, the study did suggest a possible link to attention problems; however, an additional study examining possible intellectual and behavioral effects of in-utero exposure to corticosteroids failed to demonstrate an increased risk of attention problems [45, 46].

While use of short courses of corticosteroids are considered relatively safe in pregnancy, use should be limited, especially during the first trimester. A meta-analysis examining birth defects after maternal exposure failed to show a statistically significant difference in the occurrence of major birth anomalies between exposed and unexposed groups; however, when a single study was removed from the meta-analysis, data suggested an increased risk of birth anomalies, specifically cleft lips/cleft palates, when exposure occurred during the first trimester. Additionally, a sub-analysis of all case-control studies examining incidence of cleft lips/cleft palates demonstrated a 3.4-fold increased risk in exposed groups [47]. Therefore, recommendations are for an initial dose of 0.5 ~ 2 mg/kg/day, depending on disease severity, with a maintenance dose that does not exceed 10–15 mg/day to decrease risk of cleft lips/cleft palates [23].

Of note, corticosteroids are considered safe in the breastfeeding mother given their favorable pharmacokinetic profile and can be prescribed in the post-partum period [48]. However, given drug pharmacokinetics, it is recommended that patients wait 4 hours after dosage before breastfeeding [39].

Cyclosporine

The FDA previously classified cyclosporine as pregnancy category C [5]. While cyclosporine crosses the placenta, with blood concentrations in the fetus measured at 30–64% that of maternal levels, it is considered a relatively safe medication for use in pregnancy [49]. In animal studies, fetal toxicity was only seen with maternally toxic doses of cyclosporine [49] Studies examining fetal effects of in utero cyclosporine exposure suggest an association with low birth weight and prematurity; however, the complicated health status of the patient populations studied likely confounded this association [39]. Additionally the theoretic risk of immune system dysfunction in newborns exposed to cyclosporine in utero has not been supported, with evidence in the literature refuting this theory [50]. Given its relatively favorable safety profile, cyclosporine is considered one of the best options when systemic treatments are considered for atopic dermatitis. In fact, a recent position paper by the European Task Force on Atopic Dermatitis (ETFAD) lists cyclosporine as their treatment of choice when long term therapy is required in recalcitrant or severe atopic dermatitis [13]. It is important for the prescribing provider to bear in mind that while not clearly teratogenic, cyclosporine is nephrotoxic. Thus, treatment courses should be limited to the shortest duration possible, and blood pressure and renal function monitoring is necessary in the mother while undergoing treatment [13, 22, 51]. Further, the prescribing provider should bear in mind that cyclosporine is contraindicated in breastfeeding mothers because cyclosporine is secreted in breast milk; thus, alternative treatment strategies would be needed postpartum should the patient plan to breastfeed [49, 52].

Dupilumab

There are no studies to date evaluating the safety of dupilumab in the pregnant patient. Dupilumab is an immunoglobulin G4 (IgG4) antibody against IL4alpha, a subunit present in both the IL4 and the IL13 receptor [53]. As IgG4 has the second highest transplacental transport of all antibody subtypes, it is likely that dupilumab crosses the placenta and accumulates in the fetus [54]. However, there are no data to suggest a teratogenic effect of dupilumab. There are also no data to suggest whether dupilumab leads to other complications of pregnancy such as premature birth and spontaneous abortion. Still, the mechanism of action of dupilumab, specifically blocking Th2 cytokines thought to play a role in the maintenance of pregnancy, does imply possible consequences to the fetus. In line with this, unpublished data from Piccinni et al. demonstrated reduced IL4 and IL10 production by T cell clones generated from the placenta of women with unexplained recurrent spontaneous abortions as compared to the placenta of women with voluntary abortions [11]. Thus, until more data are available to determine the safety of dupilumab in pregnancy, alternative systemic treatments with more available safety data should be favored.

Azathioprine

The FDA previously classified azathioprine as pregnancy category D [5]. The use of azathioprine in pregnancy is controversial, as it freely crosses the placenta and has been linked to preterm births, intrauterine growth restriction, miscarriage, and low birth weight [51, 55, 56]. However, these associations may be confounded by the complicated maternal health status of the patient populations studied [57]. While azathioprine may carry the above-enumerated risks, it does not appear to cause fetal anomalies, thought in large part due to the inability of the fetal liver to convert azathioprine into its active metabolites [56, 58]. Of note, no studies to date have examined the use of azathioprine in pregnant patients with atopic dermatitis. Additionally, azathioprine is secreted in breast milk and should be avoided by nursing mothers [59]. Therefore, when considering systemic medications for the pregnant woman with severe atopic dermatitis, azathioprine should only be considered when other options have failed to control severe or recalcitrant disease.

Systemic Antibiotics

In patients with extensive bacterial superinfections, providers should evaluate and treat with systemic antibiotics considered safe for use in pregnancy, including penicillins, cephalosporins and azithromycin. [41, 56] Interestingly, recent reports indicate increased risk of infantile atopic dermatitis in children born to mothers with prenatal antibiotic exposure [60, 61]. The reason for this is unclear; however, it has been suggested that antibiotic exposure modifies early gut microbiota that play an integral role in immune system development [60]. Numerous studies examining the effect of probiotics in atopic dermatitis report decreased risk of atopic dermatitis development with prenatal probiotic administration without preceding antibiotic exposure [62, 63]. However, the role for prenatal probiotic administration for prevention of atopic dermatitis remains controversial, and the ability of probiotics to counter any deleterious effects secondary to antibiotic exposure is unclear. Nonetheless, as probiotics are thought to be safe in pregnancy, providers may consider supplementation with probiotics when prescribing systemic antibiotics [64].

Acyclovir

The FDA classifies acyclovir as previous pregnancy category B. Studies support the safety of acyclovir use in pregnant and lactating patients, with no increase in infant toxicities or adverse events seen with *in utero* exposure or breastfeeding [65–67].

Antihistamines

Most systemic first generation antihistamines are former FDA pregnancy category B and considered safe for use in pregnancy [22]. However, promethazine and hydroxyzine are classified as former FDA pregnancy category C due to limited well-controlled studies demonstrating safety in human populations [68]. Additionally, in-utero exposure to hydroxyzine during the first trimester has been associated with a mildly increased risk of congenital anomalies as compared to the general population [41, 69]. While this risk has not been definitively proven, alternative first-generation antihistamines are favored in the pregnant patient. Of note, one study did find an association between diphenhydramine and risk of cleft palate; however, subsequent studies of antihistamine use in pregnancy have not corroborated this finding [70]. Further, when administered intravenously or at levels sufficient to cause overdose, diphenhydramine may cause an oxytocin-like effect, leading to uterine hyperstimulation and distress to the fetus [71, 72]. As such, low dose chlorpheniramine and diphenhydramine are preferred over other first generation antihistamines in pregnancy [5]. While the limited data on second-generation antihistamines also demonstrate no teratogenic effects, first-generation antihistamines are recommended given more extensive safety data [68]. Should first-generation antihistamines be too sedating, second-generation antihistamines can be considered. However, recent systemic reviews note no clear improvement in atopic dermatitis-associated pruritus in patients using second generation antihistamines as monotherapy or in conjunction with topical treatments [73, 74]. Animal studies examining the effect of second-generation antihistamines in pregnancy suggest no increased risk of teratogenicity with loratadine and cetirizine; however, in utero exposure to fexofenadine was associated with adverse effects to the fetus [68]. Therefore, loratadine is favored when second generation antihistamines are used in pregnancy [5, 75]. While antihistamines are regarded as safe during pregnancy, they should be used with caution in the last weeks of pregnancy, as they may cause infant withdrawal symptoms . These symptoms, including irritability, diarrhea, and grand mal seizures, may persist for up to 4 weeks after birth and are most associated with high doses of antihistamines taken during the last month of pregnancy [76, 77]. Further, a single study demonstrated an association between antihistamine use during the last 2 weeks of pregnancy and retrolental fibroplasia; however, additional studies have not corroborated this finding [78].

Of note, while first-generation antihistamines are preferred during pregnancy, second-generation antihistamines, specifically loratadine, are preferred during breast feeding as they are less sedating, are found in low levels in breast milk, and are thought to have less of an impact on breast milk production than first generation antihistamines [5].

Unsafe Agents: Methotrexate, Mycophenolate, Psoralens

Certain treatments with great utility in the non-pregnant patient should be avoided in the pregnant patient with atopic dermatitis. Methotrexate is classified as former FDA pregnancy category X as it is teratogenic and associated with numerous fetal anomalies [79]. This medication should be stopped at least 3 months prior to planned conception [5]. Mycophenolate mofetil (MMF) is a former FDA pregnancy category D and should be avoided in pregnancy given accumulating evidence suggesting teratogenicity of MMF [5, 80]. While psoralens, used in combination with UVA phototherapy (PUVA), are classified as a previous FDA pregnancy category C, the literature suggests its avoidance in pregnancy due to a theoretical risk of teratogenesis [5].

Summary

The following table summarizes the treatment options for atopic dermatitis during pregnancy. Choice of treatment depends on the severity and extent of the dermatitis, the stage of pregnancy, and whether or not secondary infection is present (Table 5.1).

Table 5.1 Treatment of atopic dermatitis during pregnancy

First-line treatment
Basic care with emollients, tepid baths, mild cleansers
Topical steroids (former FDA pregnancy category C)
Recommendations [13, 32]
Short courses preferred
Low to mid-potency preferred
Avoid fluticasone propionate
If exceeding 200 g per month, consider addition of phototherapy
Risks [29–31]
Possible association with low birth weight (low quality evidence)
Breastfeeding considerations [13]
Clean nipples before feeding
Phototherapy
Recommendations [13, 33]
UVB and UVA may be used liberally
Avoid psoralen in pregnancy
Risks [13, 35, 36]
May worsen melasma
Watch for folate deficiencies
Breastfeeding considerations [13]
Avoid psoralen in the breastfeeding woman
Second-line treatment
Systemic corticosteroids (former FDA pregnancy category C)
Recommendations [23, 47]
Recommended treatment for short term rescue therapy
Non-halogenated corticosteroids should be favored over halogenated corticosteroids
Limit use in the first trimester
Dosing should not exceed 10–15 mg/day
Risks [42–47]
Inconclusive data
Possible association with cleft palates, low birth weight, IUGR, GERD, attention problems
Breastfeeding considerations [48] [39]
Considered safe in breastfeeding woman
Recommend waiting 4 hours after dosage prior to breastfeeding
Cyclosporine (former FDA pregnancy category C)
Recommendations [13]
Recommended treatment when long-term systemic treatment is required for recalcitrant or severe disease

(continued)

Table 5.1 (continued)

Blood pressure and renal function monitoring during treatment
Risks [13, 39]
Nephrotoxic
Inconclusive data
Possible association with prematurity, low birth weight
Breastfeeding considerations [49, 52]
Contraindicated in breast feeding
Alternative/adjunctive treatments
Topical calcineurin inhibitors
Recommendations
Favor topical corticosteroids, given more safety data
Risks:
Unclear risks given limited data on topical form
Breastfeeding considerations [40]
If used in breastfeeding woman, nipple should be spared
Azathioprine (former FDA pregnancy category D)
Recommendations [13]
Consider when patient fails other systemic treatments
Risks [51, 55, 56]
Possible association with IUGR, miscarriage, low birth weight
Breastfeeding considerations [59]
Avoid in breastfeeding mother as secreted in breast milk
Dupilumab (pregnancy category – Not assigned)
Recommendations
Favor more well-studied systemic treatments
Risks:
Unknown effects in pregnant women
Breastfeeding considerations
Unknown effects in lactating women
Antihistamines (former FDA pregnancy category B and C)
Recommendations
First generation antihistamines preferred
Avoid promethazine and hydroxyzine
Favor loratadine if second generation antihistamines
Risks
Infant withdrawal symptoms if used in last weeks of pregnancy
Possible association with retrolental fibroplasia if used in final weeks of pregnancy
Breastfeeding considerations
Second generation antihistamines preferred
Interventions to avoid in pregnancy
Methotrexate (pregnancy category X)
Mycophenolate mofetil (pregnancy category D)

Conflicts of Interest Neither author has any conflict of interest to declare.

References

1. Ambros-Rudolph CM, Mullegger RR, Vaughan-Jones SA, Kerl H, Black MM. The specific dermatoses of pregnancy revisited and reclassified: results of a retrospective two-center study on 505 pregnant patients. J Am Acad Dermatol. 2006;54:395–404.
2. Vaughan Jones SA, Hern S, Nelson-Piercy C, Seed PT, Black MM. A prospective study of 200 women with dermatoses of pregnancy correlating clinical findings with hormonal and immunopathological profiles. Br J Dermatol. 1999;141:71–81.
3. Cho S, Kim HJ, Oh SH, Park CO, Jung JY, Lee KH. The influence of pregnancy and menstruation on the deterioration of atopic dermatitis symptoms. Ann Dermatol. 2010;22:180–5.
4. Kemmett D, Tidman MJ. The influence of the menstrual cycle and pregnancy on atopic dermatitis. Br J Dermatol. 1991;125:59–61.
5. Babalola O, Strober BE. Treatment of atopic dermatitis in pregnancy. Dermatol Ther. 2013;26:293–301.
6. Yang CS, Teeple M, Muglia J, Robinson-Bostom L. Inflammatory and glandular skin disease in pregnancy. Clin Dermatol. 2016;34:335–43.
7. Kroumpouzos G. Text atlas of obstetric dermatology. Philadelphia: Lippincott, Williams & Wilkins; 2014.
8. Feinberg BB, Gonik B. General precepts of the immunology of pregnancy. Clin Obstet Gynecol. 1991;34:3–16.
9. Garcia-Gonzalez E, Ahued-Ahued R, Arroyo E, Montes-De-Oca D, Granados J. Immunology of the cutaneous disorders of pregnancy. Int J Dermatol. 1999;38:721–9.
10. Haimovici F, Hill JA, Anderson DJ. The effects of soluble products of activated lymphocytes and macrophages on blastocyst implantation events in vitro. Biol Reprod. 1991;44:69–75.
11. Romagnani S. The Th1/Th2 paradigm. Immunol Today. 1997;18:263–6.
12. Eyerich K, Novak N. Immunology of atopic eczema: overcoming the Th1/Th2 paradigm. Allergy. 2013;68:974–82.
13. Vestergaard C, Wollenberg A, Barbarot S, Christen-Zaech S, Deleuran M, Spuls P, et al. European task force on atopic dermatitis position paper: treatment of parental atopic dermatitis during preconception, pregnancy and lactation period. J Eur Acad Dermatol Venereol. 2019;33:1644–59.
14. Peters EM, Michenko A, Kupfer J, Kummer W, Wiegand S, Niemeier V, et al. Mental stress in atopic dermatitis--neuronal plasticity and the cholinergic system are affected in atopic dermatitis and in response to acute experimental mental stress in a randomized controlled pilot study. PLoS One. 2014;9:e113552.
15. Hamann CR, Egeberg A, Wollenberg A, Gislason G, Skov L, Thyssen JP. Pregnancy complications, treatment characteristics and birth outcomes in women with atopic dermatitis in Denmark. J Eur Acad Dermatol Venereol. 2019;33:577–87.
16. Avgil M, Ornoy A. Herpes simplex virus and Epstein-Barr virus infections in pregnancy: consequences of neonatal or intrauterine infection. Reprod Toxicol. 2006;21:436–45.
17. Cowell WJ, Bellinger DC, Wright RO, Wright RJ. Antenatal active maternal asthma and other atopic disorders is associated with ADHD behaviors among school-aged children. Brain Behav Immun. 2019;80:871–8.
18. Thurmann L, Herberth G, Rolle-Kampczyk U, Roder S, Borte M, von Bergen M, et al. Elevated gestational IL-13 during fetal development is associated with hyperactivity and inattention in eight-year-old children. Front Immunol. 2019;10:1658.

19. El-Heis S, Crozier SR, Healy E, Robinson SM, Harvey NC, Cooper C, et al. Maternal stress and psychological distress preconception: association with offspring atopic eczema at age 12 months. Clin Exp Allergy. 2017;47:760–9.
20. Chang HY, Suh DI, Yang SI, Kang MJ, Lee SY, Lee E, et al. Prenatal maternal distress affects atopic dermatitis in offspring mediated by oxidative stress. J Allergy Clin Immunol. 2016;138:468–75. e5
21. Cork MJ, Eckert L, Simpson EL, Armstrong A, Barbarot S, Puig L, et al. Dupilumab improves patient-reported symptoms of atopic dermatitis, symptoms of anxiety and depression, and health-related quality of life in moderate-to-severe atopic dermatitis: analysis of pooled data from the randomized trials SOLO 1 and SOLO 2. J Dermatolog Treat. 2019:1–9.
22. Lehrhoff S, Pomeranz MK. Specific dermatoses of pregnancy and their treatment. Dermatol Ther. 2013;26:274–84.
23. Ambros-Rudolph CM. Dermatoses of pregnancy - clues to diagnosis, fetal risk and therapy. Ann Dermatol. 2011;23:265–75.
24. EL Leung DY, Boguniewicz M. Atopic dermatitis (atopic eczema). In: Goldsmith L, Katz SL, Gilchrest BA, Paller AS, Leffell DJ, Wolff K, editors. Fitzpatrick's dermatology in general medicine. 8th ed. New York: McGraw-Hill; 2012.
25. Papadakis MAMS, Rabow MW, Berger TG. Dermatologic disorders. In: Papadakis MA, McPhee SG, editors. Current medical diagnosis & treatment. 52nd ed. New York: McGraw-Hill Professional Publishing; 2013.
26. Edwards MJ, Agho K, Attia J, Diaz P, Hayes T, Illingworth A, et al. Case-control study of cleft lip or palate after maternal use of topical corticosteroids during pregnancy. Am J Med Genet A. 2003;120A:459–63.
27. Czeizel AE, Rockenbauer M. Population-based case-control study of teratogenic potential of corticosteroids. Teratology. 1997;56:335–40.
28. Carmichael SL, Shaw GM, Ma C, Werler MM, Rasmussen SA, Lammer EJ, et al. Maternal corticosteroid use and orofacial clefts. Am J Obstet Gynecol. 2007;197:585 e1–7; discussion 683–4, e1–7.
29. Mygind H, Thulstrup AM, Pedersen L, Larsen H. Risk of intrauterine growth retardation, malformations and other birth outcomes in children after topical use of corticosteroid in pregnancy. Acta Obstet Gynecol Scand. 2002;81:234–9.
30. Hviid A, Molgaard-Nielsen D. Corticosteroid use during pregnancy and risk of orofacial clefts. CMAJ. 2011;183:796–804.
31. Chi CC, Wang SH, Wojnarowska F, Kirtschig G, Davies E, Bennett C. Safety of topical corticosteroids in pregnancy. Cochrane Database Syst Rev. 2015:CD007346.
32. Chi CC, Kirtschig G, Aberer W, Gabbud JP, Lipozencic J, Karpati S, et al. Evidence-based (S3) guideline on topical corticosteroids in pregnancy. Br J Dermatol. 2011;165:943–52.
33. Wollenberg A, Ehmann LM. Long term treatment concepts and proactive therapy for atopic eczema. Ann Dermatol. 2012;24:253–60.
34. Darsow U, Wollenberg A, Simon D, Taieb A, Werfel T, Oranje A, et al. ETFAD/EADV eczema task force 2009 position paper on diagnosis and treatment of atopic dermatitis. J Eur Acad Dermatol Venereol. 2010;24:317–28.
35. Lam J, Polifka JE, Dohil MA. Safety of dermatologic drugs used in pregnant patients with psoriasis and other inflammatory skin diseases. J Am Acad Dermatol. 2008;59:295–315.
36. Park KK, Murase JE. Narrowband UV-B phototherapy during pregnancy and folic acid depletion. Arch Dermatol. 2012;148:132–3.
37. Jain AB, Reyes J, Marcos A, Mazariegos G, Eghtesad B, Fontes PA, et al. Pregnancy after liver transplantation with tacrolimus immunosuppression: a single center's experience update at 13 years. Transplantation. 2003;76:827–32.
38. Kainz A, Harabacz I, Cowlrick IS, Gadgil SD, Hagiwara D. Review of the course and outcome of 100 pregnancies in 84 women treated with tacrolimus. Transplantation. 2000;70:1718–21.
39. Bae YS, Van Voorhees AS, Hsu S, Korman NJ, Lebwohl MG, Young M, et al. Review of treatment options for psoriasis in pregnant or lactating women: from the medical Board of the National Psoriasis Foundation. J Am Acad Dermatol. 2012;67:459–77.

40. Gardiner SJ, Begg EJ. Breastfeeding during tacrolimus therapy. Obstet Gynecol. 2006;107:453–5.
41. Briggs GGFR, Yaffe SJ. Drugs in pregnancy and lactation: a reference guide to fetal and neonatal risk. Philadelphia: Lippincot Williams & Wilkins; 2008.
42. Chin SO, Brodsky NL, Bhandari V. Antenatal steroid use is associated with increased gastroesophageal reflux in neonates. Am J Perinatol. 2003;20:205–13.
43. Gur C, Diav-Citrin O, Shechtman S, Arnon J, Ornoy A. Pregnancy outcome after first trimester exposure to corticosteroids: a prospective controlled study. Reprod Toxicol. 2004;18:93–101.
44. Wapner RJ, Sorokin Y, Mele L, Johnson F, Dudley DJ, Spong CY, et al. Long-term outcomes after repeat doses of antenatal corticosteroids. N Engl J Med. 2007;357:1190–8.
45. Crowther CA, Doyle LW, Haslam RR, Hiller JE, Harding JE, Robinson JS, et al. Outcomes at 2 years of age after repeat doses of antenatal corticosteroids. N Engl J Med. 2007;357:1179–89.
46. Schmand B, Neuvel J, Smolders-de Haas H, Hoeks J, Treffers PE, Koppe JG. Psychological development of children who were treated antenatally with corticosteroids to prevent respiratory distress syndrome. Pediatrics. 1990;86:58–64.
47. Park-Wyllie L, Mazzotta P, Pastuszak A, Moretti ME, Beique L, Hunnisett L, et al. Birth defects after maternal exposure to corticosteroids: prospective cohort study and meta-analysis of epidemiological studies. Teratology. 2000;62:385–92.
48. Greenberger PA, Odeh YK, Frederiksen MC, Atkinson AJ Jr. Pharmacokinetics of prednisolone transfer to breast milk. Clin Pharmacol Ther. 1993;53:324–8.
49. Briggs GG, Freeman RK, Yaffe SJ. Cyclosporine. In: Briggs GG, Freeman RK, Yaffe SJ, editors. Drugs in Pregnancy and Lactation. 9th ed. Philadelphia: Lippincott Williams and Wilkins; 2011. p. 351–3.
50. Motta M, Ciardelli L, Marconi M, Tincani A, Gasparoni A, Lojacono A, et al. Immune system development in infants born to mothers with autoimmune disease, exposed in utero to immunosuppressive agents. Am J Perinatol. 2007;24:441–7.
51. Koutroulis I, Papoutsis J, Kroumpouzos G. Atopic dermatitis in pregnancy: current status and challenges. Obstet Gynecol Surv. 2011;66:654–63.
52. American Academy of Pediatrics Committee on Drugs. Transfer of drugs and other chemicals into human milk. Pediatrics. 2001;108:776–89.
53. Seegraber M, Srour J, Walter A, Knop M, Wollenberg A. Dupilumab for treatment of atopic dermatitis. Expert Rev Clin Pharmacol. 2018;11:467–74.
54. Koren G, Ornoy A. The role of the placenta in drug transport and fetal drug exposure. Expert Rev Clin Pharmacol. 2018;11:373–85.
55. Tendron A, Gouyon JB, Decramer S. In utero exposure to immunosuppressive drugs: experimental and clinical studies. Pediatr Nephrol. 2002;17:121–30.
56. Weatherhead S, Robson SC, Reynolds NJ. Eczema in pregnancy. BMJ. 2007;335:152–4.
57. Cleary BJ, Kallen B. Early pregnancy azathioprine use and pregnancy outcomes. Birth Defects Res A Clin Mol Teratol. 2009;85:647–54.
58. Janssen NM, Genta MS. The effects of immunosuppressive and anti-inflammatory medications on fertility, pregnancy, and lactation. Arch Intern Med. 2000;160:610–9.
59. Habal FM, Huang VW. Review article: a decision-making algorithm for the management of pregnancy in the inflammatory bowel disease patient. Aliment Pharmacol Ther. 2012;35:501–15.
60. Timm S, Schlunssen V, Olsen J, Ramlau-Hansen CH. Prenatal antibiotics and atopic dermatitis among 18-month-old children in the Danish National Birth Cohort. Clin Exp Allergy. 2017;47:929–36.
61. Lee SY, Yu J, Ahn KM, Kim KW, Shin YH, Lee KS, et al. Additive effect between IL-13 polymorphism and cesarean section delivery/prenatal antibiotics use on atopic dermatitis: a birth cohort study (COCOA). PLoS One. 2014;9:e96603.
62. Ro ADB, Simpson MR, Ro TB, Storro O, Johnsen R, Videm V, et al. Reduced Th22 cell proportion and prevention of atopic dermatitis in infants following maternal probiotic supplementation. Clin Exp Allergy. 2017;47:1014–21.

63. Rautava S, Kainonen E, Salminen S, Isolauri E. Maternal probiotic supplementation during pregnancy and breast-feeding reduces the risk of eczema in the infant. J Allergy Clin Immunol. 2012;130:1355–60.
64. Elias J, Bozzo P, Einarson A. Are probiotics safe for use during pregnancy and lactation? Can Fam Physician. 2011;57:299–301.
65. Latta RA, Baker DA. Treatment of recurrent eczema herpeticum in pregnancy with acyclovir. Infect Dis Obstet Gynecol. 1996;4:239–42.
66. Drake AL, Roxby AC, Kiarie J, Richardson BA, Wald A, John-Stewart G, et al. Infant safety during and after maternal valacyclovir therapy in conjunction with antiretroviral HIV-1 prophylaxis in a randomized clinical trial. PLoS One. 2012;7(4):e34635.
67. Pasternak B, Hviid A. Use of acyclovir, valacyclovir, and famciclovir in the first trimester of pregnancy and the risk of birth defects. JAMA. 2010;304:859–66.
68. Kar S, Krishnan A, Preetha K, Mohankar A. A review of antihistamines used during pregnancy. J Pharmacol Pharmacother. 2012;3:105–8.
69. Tang Y, Ma CX, Cui W, Chang V, Ariet M, Morse SB, et al. The risk of birth defects in multiple births: a population-based study. Matern Child Health J. 2006;10:75–81.
70. Saxen I. Letter: cleft palate and maternal diphenhydramine intake. Lancet. 1974;1:407–8.
71. Brost BC, Scardo JA, Newman RB. Diphenhydramine overdose during pregnancy: lessons from the past. Am J Obstet Gynecol. 1996;175:1376–7.
72. Hara GS, Carter RP, Krantz KE. Dramamine in labor: potential boon or a possible bomb? J Kans Med Soc. 1980;81:134–6. 55
73. Matterne U, Bohmer MM, Weisshaar E, Jupiter A, Carter B, Apfelbacher CJ. Oral H1 antihistamines as 'add-on' therapy to topical treatment for eczema. Cochrane Database Syst Rev. 2019;1:CD012167.
74. van Zuuren EJ, Apfelbacher CJ, Fedorowicz Z, Jupiter A, Matterne U, Weisshaar E. No high level evidence to support the use of oral H1 antihistamines as monotherapy for eczema: a summary of a Cochrane systematic review. Syst Rev. 2014;3:25.
75. Diav-Citrin O, Shechtman S, Aharonovich A, Moerman L, Arnon J, Wajnberg R, et al. Pregnancy outcome after gestational exposure to loratadine or antihistamines: a prospective controlled cohort study. J Allergy Clin Immunol. 2003;111:1239–43.
76. Lione A, Scialli AR. The developmental toxicity of the H1 histamine antagonists. Reprod Toxicol. 1996;10:247–55.
77. Serreau R, Komiha M, Blanc F, Guillot F, Jacqz-Aigrain E. Neonatal seizures associated with maternal hydroxyzine hydrochloride in late pregnancy. Reprod Toxicol. 2005;20:573–4.
78. Purohit DM, Ellison RC, Zierler S, Miettinen OS, Nadas AS. Risk factors for retrolental fibroplasia: experience with 3,025 premature infants. National Collaborative Study on patent Ductus arteriosus in premature infants. Pediatrics. 1985;76:339–44.
79. Hyoun SC, Obican SG, Scialli AR. Teratogen update: methotrexate. Birth Defects Res A Clin Mol Teratol. 2012;94:187–207.
80. Tyler KH. Dermatologic therapy in pregnancy. Clin Obstet Gynecol. 2015;58:112–8.

Chapter 6
Acne and Rosacea in Pregnancy

Casey A. Spell, Hannah R. Badon, Amy Flischel, and Robert T. Brodell

Introduction

The management of acne or rosacea during pregnancy is complex. Challenges include the potential for fetal toxicity, discrepancies in safety data, and the paucity of evidence-based treatment guidelines [1]. Nevertheless, safe treatment options are available, and effective regimens can be designed for pregnant patients. This chapter considers the pathophysiology, diagnosis, and treatment of acne and rosacea, focusing on patients presenting before, during, and after pregnancy.

Cutaneous Changes During Pregnancy

Pregnancy is associated with a myriad of physiologic changes that affect essentially every organ system in the body. The integument is no exception. The cutaneous changes that occur during pregnancy are modulated by complex "cross talk" between hormonal, immunologic, and metabolic mediators [2, 3]. The resultant

Author Attribution Casey Spell and Hannah Badon wrote the first draft of this manuscript. Robert T. Brodell, MD, reviewed and approved the content of this manuscript.

C. A. Spell (✉)
University of Mississippi Medical School, Jackson, MS, USA
e-mail: cspell@umc.edu

H. R. Badon · R. T. Brodell
Department of Dermatology, University of Mississippi Medical Center, Jackson, MS, USA

A. Flischel
Northwestern Medical Group, Vernon Hills, IL, USA

K. H. Tyler (ed.), *Cutaneous Disorders of Pregnancy*,
https://doi.org/10.1007/978-3-030-49285-4_6

inflammatory and glandular skin changes are associated with a gradual shift from cell-mediated to humoral immune responses throughout gestation. This switch from Type 1 T helper cells (Th1) to a predominance of Type 2 T helper cells (Th2) is thought to play a critical role in placental immune tolerance. This immunologic adjustment comes with a tradeoff leading to a worsening of conditions involving sebaceous and eccrine glands, while diseases of the apocrine glands tend to improve. Of course, not all pregnancies follow these general trends [4]. While 90% of women experience skin changes during pregnancy, acne and rosacea are among the most distressing [3, 5].

Acne

Epidemiology

Acne has a prevalence ranging from 85–100% in adolescence [6, 7]. While many patients experience a regression of acne after their teenage years, others have symptoms that can persist well into adulthood [6]. Despite acne's being so common, only a few studies have focused on acne treatment during pregnancy.

In one French study, 42.3% of 378 pregnant patients examined by dermatologists were found to have acne. Among these acne patients, 86.6% reported having acne prior to pregnancy, while another 35.1% reported a relapse of previously "cured" acne during pregnancy. Another 51.5% reported unremitting acne since adolescence. Among all surveyed patients, 59.7% reported worsening acne symptoms, 9.1% improving symptoms, and 31.2% no change in symptoms through the course of pregnancy [8]. The clinical course of acne in pregnancy is variable, and reports are not consistent across other studies [9].

Pathophysiology

Acne vulgaris is a chronic inflammatory disorder of the pilosebaceous unit [6]. Triggers include: the upregulation of androgens, increased sebum production, follicular hyperkeratinization, inflammatory processes, dietary influences, and overgrowth of facial microbiota such as *Propionibacterium acnes (P. acnes)*. It is unclear which of these factors, or combination of factors, is responsible for the exacerbation of acne during pregnancy, but hormonal modulation at the level of the sebaceous gland likely plays a significant role [9].

Hormonal fluctuations during pregnancy have a profound effect on activity within the sebaceous glands. Estrogen, progesterone, and human chorionic gonadotropin (hCG) lead to cutaneous changes which peak during the first and third trimesters. The upregulation of hCG in early pregnancy promotes the production of estrogen and progesterone, both of which increase until the time of delivery. Progesterone has been most commonly linked to acne during pregnancy, especially in women with increased insulin resistance, i.e. patients with polycystic ovarian syndrome (PCOS) and a prior diagnosis of diabetes [10, 11]. The presence of excess insulin also stimulates the growth and maturation of the sebaceous glands, a process mediated by the upregulation of growth hormone (GH) receptors on sebocytes. Furthermore, insulin downregulates sex hormone binding globulin (SHBG) in the liver, and this has a positive feedback on adrenal and ovarian androgenesis [12]. Thus, increased levels of serum insulin during pregnancy lead to androgen excess and sebum production.

Increases, decreases, or disruptions in sebum production have been associated with the pathophysiology of acne vulgaris [13]. Sebum is closely tied to the body's production of androgens such as 5α-dihydrotestosterone (5α-DHT). Increases in androgens inside the pilosebaceous unit or increased sensitivity of the unit can lead to the release of sebum and possible acne exacerbation.

Diagnosis

The diagnosis of acne is made by physical examination. Patients present with closed comedones (whiteheads), open comedones (blackheads), papules, pustules, and cysts. Differential diagnosis of acne vulgaris includes perioral dermatitis, rosacea, milia, and keratosis pilaris rubra faceii. Typically, bacterial cultures are negative but, on occasion, a gram negative bacteria may be identified, especially in patients not responding to antibiotic treatment. Serologic testing is generally not performed for acne patients unless polycystic ovarian syndrome is suspected or if patients have a history of oligomenorrhea, hirsutism, acanthosis nigricans, or a family history of hyperandrogenism. In these patients, total and free testosterone, dehydroepiandrosterone sulfate (DHEAS), androstenedione, luteinizing hormone, and follicle-stimulating hormone, as well as a lipid panel, glucose, and insulin level can be obtained [14].

Treatment

Acne treatment involves topical, oral, and physical therapies. Some of these options are limited in pregnant patients. In one study, pregnant patients were most commonly treated with topical antibiotics (53.5%), oral zinc gluconate 30 mg/day (89.9%), and no prescription (5.6%) [8]. Selected systemic antibiotics can also be utilized with an effort to minimize the risk of harm to mother and fetus.

Safety Profile of Common Acne Medications in Pregnancy

Topical agents are considered first line in pregnant patients with acne. Systemic therapies may be utilized in more severe or refractory acne. Very little research exists regarding cosmetic procedures during pregnancy.

A system whereby the Federal Drug Administraion (FDA) assigned a letter category (A,B,C,D, and X) to each drug (Table 6.1) was replaced by a narrative system focusing on specified information required in the package insert of each prescription drug (Table 6.2) [9]. The new system, unfortunately, requires a high

Table 6.1 "Classic" US Food and Drug Administration (FDA) Drug Risk Classification System for Pregnant Women

Category	Definition
A	Adequate and well-controlled human studies have failed to demonstrate a risk to the fetus in the first trimester of pregnancy (and there is no evidence of risk in later trimesters)
B	Animal reproduction studies have failed to demonstrate a risk to the fetus and there are no adequate and well-controlled studies in pregnant women OR animal studies have shown an adverse effect, but adequate and well-controlled studies have failed to demonstrate a risk to the fetus in any trimester
C	Animal reproduction studies have shown an adverse effect on the fetus and there are no adequate and well-controlled studies in humans, but potential benefits may warrant use of the drug in women despite potential risks
D	There is positive evidence of human fetal risks based on adverse reaction data from investigational or marketing experience or studies in humans, but potential benefits may warrant use of the drug in pregnant women despite potential risks
X	Studies in animals or humans have demonstrated fetal abnormalities and/or there is evidence of human fetal risk based on adverse reaction data from investigational or marketing experience and the risks involved in the use of the drug in pregnant women clearly outweigh potential benefits

Table 6.2 New Narrative FDA System Describing Safety of Drugs During Pregnancy and Lactation

Pregnancy (includes labor and delivery):
Pregnancy exposure registry
Risk summary
Clinical considerations
Data
Lactation (includes nursing mothers)
Risk summary
Clinical considerations
Data
Females and males of reproductive potential
Pregnancy testing
Contraception
Infertility

level of decision making expertise when compared to the older system. Furthermore, as of 2015, older medications and over-the-counter products approved prior to June 30, 2001 have neither a pregnancy category nor a narrative summary. The close collaboration required between the FDA and manufacturers to ensure timely updates is also problematic. In addition, consumers may not adequately cooperate by sharing their health information with pregnancy registries to accumulate a meaningful amount of data [15, 16]. Finally, patients can be confused by the new system that eliminates simple categories defining risk. We have chosen to use the older categories along with a narrative description in this chapter. Providers should refer to prescription package inserts for additional safety information.

Topical Treatment Options

1. Azelaic Acid

Azelaic acid is a former FDA pregnancy category B medication. It is a dicarboxylic acid with antimicrobial and anti-inflammatory properties used to suppress the formation of microcomedones and improve acne [17, 18]. In addition, it is an inhibitor of tyrosinase, which can reduce hyperpigmentation. It has also been known to cause a transient burning sensation in some patients [19]. Animal studies indicate no adverse birth outcomes, and less than 4% of applied medication is systemically absorbed [20]. Azelaic acid is also found in several foods including milk, barley, rye, and wheat. This drug is considered a safe choice for topical acne treatment during pregnancy [18, 19].

2. Benzoyl Peroxide

Benzoyl peroxide (BPO) is a topical preparation with antimicrobial properties produced as a lotion, gel, wash, cream, and pledgets in concentrations ranging from 2.5 to 10%. It is a former FDA pregnancy category C medication that is commonly used in pregnancy. However, adequate safety data in pregnant patients is not available, and we advise patients to avoid applying BPO over large surfaces of skin to minimize systemic absorption [18, 20].

3. Salicylic Acid

Salicylic acid is a former FDA pregnancy category C medication that provides comedolytic and anti-inflammatory properties [18]. Systemic use is typically contraindicated during the third trimester of pregnancy due to a risk of oligohydramnios and early closure of the ductus arteriosus. Topical preparations have a systemic absorption somewhere between 9 and 25%. Pregnant patients should be advised to avoid using salicylic acid over large surface areas or under occlusive dressings to minimize systemic absorption [20]. Patients should also be informed that this is a common ingredient in many non-prescription acne washes.

4. Glycolic Acid

Glycolic acid is an α-hydroxy acid with comedolytic and keratolytic activity and can decrease sebum production [21]. The lack of an FDA pregnancy rating and definitive safety studies should limit the use of this drug, though birth complications have not been reported [18, 19].

5. Sodium Sulfacetamide

Topical sodium sulfacetamide is a bacteriostatic and anti-inflammatory agent that inhibits dihydropteroate synthetase and was previously considered FDA pregnancy category C [18]. Although sulfur-containing ointments are occasionally used by pregnant patients, a pregnancy category was never assigned by the FDA [22]. Sodium sulfacetamide lacks adequate data to support or dispute its use during pregnancy [20].

6. Topical Antibiotics

Topical antibiotic agents with both bactericidal and anti-inflammatory activity are used during pregnancy to combat the putative cause of acne: *P. acnes* [18]. Topical erythromycin and clindamycin are previous FDA pregnancy category B medications and are generally considered to be safe for use during pregnancy. Antibiotic resistance of *P. acnes* can occur when these agents are used as monotherapy. Metronidazole is another former FDA category B medication that can be safely used in pregnant patients. It has anti-inflammatory and immunosuppressive effects in addition to antimicrobial properties. Studies of metronidazole have revealed no association with adverse birth outcomes [23]. Topical dapsone is a former FDA pregnancy category C medication. It has been used during pregnancy to treat leprosy and dermatitis herpetiformis with no reports of birth defects in current literature. Oral dapsone has also been used in cases of nodulocystic acne [24]. However, a theoretical risk exists for neonatal hyperbilirubinemia when used near delivery. Any physician prescribing topical dapsone should consider stopping this regimen at least one month before delivery. Lastly, tetracycline as a topical acne preparation is contraindicated in pregnancy [20].

7. Topical Retinoids

Topical retinoids such as tretinoin and adapalene were previously categorized as FDA pregnancy category C medications. While the percutaneous absorption of tretinoin is minimal and does not alter endogenous drug levels, treatment with topical tretinoin is not recommended since this drug can cross the placenta. There have been a total of only four reports of birth defects associated with first trimester use including ear anomalies, limb reduction, and central nervous system abnormalities. In one study, 133 pregnant patients exposed to tretinoin during the first trimester showed no statistically significant increase in minor or major birth defects [25]. Adapalene is associated with rare reports of teratogenicity with exposure during the first trimester. Neither tretinoin nor adapalene has been associated with an increased risk in birth defects during the second and third trimesters. Topical tazarotene was assigned an FDA pregnancy category X due to retinoid-like anomalies found in animal studies, so this agent is contraindicated in pregnancy and lactation [20].

Systemic Treatment Options

1. Antibiotics

Commonly prescribed as second line therapy for acne, systemic antibiotics are often utilized in non-pregnant patients including tetracyclines, penicillins, macrolides (erythromycin and clindamycin), and cephalosporins [18]. Tetracyclines are considered a former FDA pregnancy category D medication and should be avoided during pregnancy, especially after 14 weeks gestation. These antibiotics deposit in the bones and teeth during the second and third trimester resulting in enamel hypoplasia and yellow staining of the teeth that may darken over time. Tetracyclines have also been associated with cases of acute fatty liver disease in mothers during the third trimester. First trimester use of tetracyclines have not been linked to congenital anomalies if medication is discontinued when pregnancy is suspected. Erythromycin, a macrolide, is a previous FDA pregnancy category B medication when used systemically; however, rare cases of hepatotoxicity have been documented with prolonged use of erythromycin ethylsuccinate. In addition, a set of Swedish studies have noted malformations in the cardiovascular system when erythromycin was used in early pregnancy. Other options that are considered safe for use during late pregnancy are azithromycin, penicillins, and cephalosporins, each of which was previously designated FDA pregnancy category B [20].

2. Spironolactone

Spironolactone is a systemic treatment used off-label to treat acne and is a previous FDA pregnancy category C medication. This drug competitively inhibits 5α-reductase and aldosterone and has been documented to cause feminization in male rat fetuses as well as delayed sexual maturation of female rat fetuses. Though these studies were not conducted in humans, spironolactone poses a high theoretical risk and should be avoided during pregnancy or in those planning for pregnancy [20].

3. Isotretinoin

Isotretinoin is a former FDA pregnancy category X medication and should never be used in pregnant or lactating patients [20]. This medication is a proven teratogen that can lead to spontaneous abortion and congenital malformations including central nervous system and thymic defects, microtia, stenosis of the external auditory canal, hydrocephalus, facial and palatal defects, and cardiovascular defects [9, 20, 26]. It is recommended that women trying to conceive stop the use of prescription retinoids for at least 1 month prior to conception [9]. Isotretinoin should not be prescribed to patients who are trying to conceive or have the potential to become pregnant.

The I-Pledge program is compulsory in the United States and is designed to ensure that no woman is prescribed oral isotretinoin without understanding its teratogenic effects. Two approved forms of contraception must be utilized while a patient is taking the prescription, and monthly pregnancy tests are required.

4. Hormone Treatment

Hormonal therapy, including oral contraceptives and androgen receptor blockers, can be useful in non-pregant patients presenting with hyperandrogenism. This therapy, however, is not recommended in pregnant patients and has been associated with an increased incidence of Down Syndrome when used in early pregnancy [27]. Anti-androgen therapy has also been associated with risks of hypospadias and feminization of the male fetus [28].

5. Zinc

Oral zinc salts have been shown to be effective in the treatment of mild to moderate cases of acne vulgaris either as monotherapy or as an adjunct to other acne treatments in dosages of 30–150 mg/day [29, 30]. Studies have shown that elemental zinc does not harm the growing fetus in dosages below 75 mg/day. In addition, no adverse effects have been reported with the use of zinc salts during lactation [31].

Cosmetic Treatment

1. Phototherapy

Narrowband (NBUVB) and broadband (BBUVB) ultraviolet B phototherapy are considered safe options for treatment during pregnancy based on data from treatment of pregnant psoriasis patients [32]. However, more recent studies have shown that cumulative exposure to NBUVB can decrease serum folic acid levels required to support the development of the fetal nervous system and prevent neural tube defects [33]. Given that folic acid requirements increase during pregnancy, it may be prudent to ensure folic acid supplementation and even perhaps monitor folic acid levels in pregnant patients treated with UV therapy [18].

2. Lasers

Fractionated CO_2 lasers for pitted acne scarring or vascular lesion lasers (595 nm) for telangiectasias should be safe during pregnancy and lactation but are generally avoided until after delivery, as are most elective treatments. Several studies reference the use of CO_2 lasers for the treatment of genital condyloma during pregnancy with no maternal or fetal complications reported [34].

Rosacea

Epidemiology

Rosacea is one of the most common dermatoses of adults. It typically presents between ages 30–50 and is especially prominent in patients of Northern European origin [35]. As with acne, there is a limited data set related to the clinical course and treatment of rosacea during pregnancy.

Rosacea fulminans (RF), or pyoderma faciale, is a rare form of rosacea that presents during pregnancy. The severe facial inflammation, numerous pustules, cystic lesions, and coalescing sinuses of RF were associated with varied obstetric outcomes in three patients: intrauterine death, termination, and routine vaginal delivery [36]. Rosacea fulminans is a possible indication for the use of topical and/or systemic corticosteroids [37]. Ocular perforation culminating from severe ocular involvement of RF was also noted in one case [38]. Treatment, therapeutic efficacy, as well as maternal and fetal outcomes are highly variable in reported cases.

Pathophysiology

The pathogenesis of rosacea may involve altered innate immunity, neurogenic inflammation, neurovascular dysregulation, and sun damage [39]. Triggers include: ultraviolet radiation, extreme temperatures, stress, spicy food, and the modulation of toll-like receptors (TLR) by various microbes [35]. More recently, demodex mites have been identified in the inflamed follicles of patients with rosacea [40]. An underlying inflammatory process within the pilosebaceous unit and facial vasculature ultimately leads to the characteristic phenotype seen in rosacea patients.

The inflammatory cascade of rosacea is tied to a molecular network of cytokines and chemokines. Toll-like receptor 2 (TLR2) signaling potentiates the release of Tumor Necrosis Factor (TNF)α and Interleukin (IL)1 which stimulate keratinocytes and leads to the recruitment of Th1 and Th17 T helper cells. These cells release other cytokines including IL17, which promotes angiogenesis via induction of vascular endothelial growth factor (VEGF). Furthermore, UV radiation (sun damage) activates keratinocyte production of Chemokine Ligand (CXCL)1 and CXCL8, facilitating neutrophil recruitment. These proposed mechanisms can explain the histopathology and phenotypic characteristic of patients with rosacea [35].

Diagnosis

Rosacea is a chronic inflammatory disease of the centrofacial skin that demonstrates a high density of sebaceous glands. Primary features of rosacea include flushing (transient erythema), chronic erythema, telangiectasias, papules, and pustules. Secondary features can include burning and stinging, plaques, dry appearance, edema, or phymatous changes.

There are four subtypes of rosacea: erythematotelangiectatic, papulopustular, phymatous, and ocular. Erythematotelangiectatic rosacea demonstrates flushing and central facial erythema. Features typically include edema, stinging and burning, roughness, and scaling dermatoses. Papulopustular rosacea presents with persistent and chronic erythema with transient papules and pustules. Phymatous rosacea demonstrates skin thickening, irregular nodularities, and enlargement. This subtype most commonly affects the nose (rhinophyma), but the forehead, chin, cheeks, and ears can show similar thickening. Ocular rosacea is the fourth subtype and can compromise vision if not treated effectively. When ocular involvement occurs, patients may present with dryness, irritation, blepharitis, conjunctivitis, or keratitis [35].

Treatment

Similar to the management of acne, the mainstay of treatment for rosacea during pregnancy is the use of selected oral and topical antibiotics. Avoidance of common clinical triggers is recommended. For cases of papulopustular rosacea, azelaic acid as well as topical antibiotics including metronidazole and clindamycin are frequently used [18]. Vascular lesion lasers (595 nm) are recommended for erythematotelangiectatic rosacea but are typically delayed until after pregnancy. Ocular rosacea can be treated with erythromycin ophthalmic ointment and sulfa eye drops [4]. Cases of rosacea fulminans during pregnancy have been treated with oral erythromycin and corticosteroids or systemic azithromycin and topical metronidazole [4, 41].

Conflict of Interest Robert T. Brodell, M.D., discloses the following potential conflicts of interest: MULTI-CENTER CLINICAL TRIALS: Genentech, Janssen Pharmaceuticals, Corrona Psoriasis Registry, Novartis, and Glaxo-Smith-Kline. Casey Spell, Hannah Badon and Amy Flischel have no conflicts of interest.

References

1. Awan SZ, Lu J. Management of severe acne during pregnancy: a case report and review of the literature. Int J Womens Dermatol. 2017;3:145–50. https://doi.org/10.1016/j.ijwd.2017.06.001.
2. Panicker VV, Riyaz N, Balachandran PK. A clinical study of cutaneous changes in pregnancy. J Epidemiol Glob Health. 2017;7:63–70. https://doi.org/10.1016/j.jegh.2016.10.002.

3. Muzaffar F, Hussain I, Haroon TS. Physiologic skin changes during pregnancy: a study of 140 cases. Int J Dermatol. 1998;37:429–31.
4. Yang CS, Teeple M, Muglia J, Robinson-Bostom L. Inflammatory and glandular skin disease in pregnancy. Clin Dermatol. 2016;34(3):335–43. https://doi.org/10.1016/j.clindermatol.2016.02.005.
5. Vora RV, Gupta R, Mehta MJ, Chaudhari AH, Pilani AP, Patel N. Pregnancy and skin. J Family Med Prim Care. 2014;3(4):318–24. https://doi.org/10.4103/2249-4863.148099.
6. Masterson KN. Acne basics: pathophysiology, assessment, and standard treatment options. J Dermatol Nurses Assoc. 2018;10:2–10. https://doi.org/10.1097/jdn.0000000000000361.
7. Meredith FM, Ormerod AD. The management of acne vulgaris in pregnancy. Am J Clin Dermatol. 2013;14:351–8. https://doi.org/10.1007/s40257-013-0041-9.
8. Dreno B, Blouin E, Moyse D, Bodokh I, Knol AC, Khammari A. Acne in pregnant women: a French survey. Acta Derm Venereol. 2014;94(1):82–3. https://doi.org/10.2340/00015555-1594.
9. Pugashetti R, Shinkai K. Treatment of acne vulgaris in pregnant patients. Dermatol Ther. 2013;26(4):302–11. https://doi.org/10.1111/dth.12077.
10. Kalanick B. What to expect from your hormones when you're expecting. 2019. Girls Gone Strong Website. https://www.girlsgonestrong.com/blog/pregnancy/pregnancy-hormones/. Accessed 15 Dec 2019.
11. Sonagra AD, Biradar SM, Dattatreya K, Murthy J. Normal pregnancy – a state of insulin resistance. J Clin Diagn Res. 2014;8(11):CC01–3. https://doi.org/10.7860/JCDR/2014/10068.5081.
12. Elsaie ML. Hormonal treatment of acne vulgaris: an update. Clin Cosmet Investig Dermatol. 2016;9:241–8. https://doi.org/10.2147/CCID.S114830.
13. Zouboulis CC. Acne and sebaceous gland function. Clin Dermatol. 2004;22(5):360–6. https://doi.org/10.1016/j.clindermatol.2004.03.004.
14. The American College of Obstetricians and Gynecologists. Routine Tests During Pregnancy. 2019. https://www.acog.org/Patients/FAQs/Routine-Tests-During-Pregnancy?IsMobileSet=false. Accessed 23 Dec 2019.
15. Pernia S, DeMaagd G. The new pregnancy and lactation labeling rule. Pregnancy and Therapeutics: P&T. 2016;41(11):713–5. PMCID: PMC5083079.
16. Beroukhim K, Abrouk M, Farahnik B. Impact of the pregnancy and lactation labeling rule (PLLR) on practicing dermatologists. Dermatol Online J. 2015;21(11):13030/qt46c4m2tw.
17. Gollnick HP, Zouboulis CC. Not all acne is acne vulgaris. Dtsch Arztebl Int. 2014;111:301–12. https://doi.org/10.3238/arztebl.2014.0301.
18. Kaptanoglu AF, Mullaaziz D. Acneiform eruptions and pregnancy. In: Acne and Acneiform eruptions; 2017. https://www.intechopen.com/books/acne-and-acneiform-eruptions/acneiform-eruptions-and-pregnancy. https://doi.org/10.5772/67015. Accessed 24 Nov 2019.
19. Zaenglein AL, Graber E, Thiboutot DM. Acne vulgaris and acneiform eruptions. In: Fitzpatrick's dermatology in general medicine; 2012. p. 8e. https://www.scribd.com/document/318288689/Fitzpatricks-Dermatology-in-General-Medicine-8Ed. Accessed 10 Dec 2019.
20. Tyler KH, Zirwas MJ. Pregnancy and dermatologic therapy. J Am Acad Dermatol. 2013;68(4):663–71. https://doi.org/10.1016/j.jaad.2012.09.034.
21. Kaminaka C, Uede M, Matsunaka H, Furukawa F, Yamomoto Y. Clinical evaluation of glycolic acid chemical peeling in patients with acne vulgaris: a randomized, double-blind, placebo-controlled, split-face comparative study. Dermatol Surg. 2014;40(3):314–22. https://doi.org/10.1111/dsu.12417.
22. Drugs.com. Sulfur Topical Pregnancy and Breastfeeding Warnings. 2019. https://www.drugs.com/pregnancy/sulfur-topical.html. Accessed 10 Dec 2019.
23. Koss CA, Baras DC, Lane SD, Aubry R, Marcus M, Markowitz LE, et al. Investigation of metronidazole use during pregnancy and adverse birth outcomes. Antimicrob Agents Chemother. 2012;56(9):4800–5. https://doi.org/10.1128/AAC.06477-11.
24. Didona D, Paolino G, Donati P, Muscardin LM. Resolution of nodulocystic acne with oral dapsone. Dermatol Ther. 2016;30(1). https://doi.org/10.1111/dth.12406.

25. Wilmer E, Chai S, Kroumpouzos G. Drug safety: pregnancy rating classifications and controversies. Clin Dermatol. 2016;34(3):401–9. https://doi.org/10.1016/j.clindermatol.2016.02.013.
26. Wolverton SE, Harper JC. Important controversies associated with isotretinoin therapy for acne. Am J Clin Dermatol. 2013;14(2):71–6. https://doi.org/10.1007/s40257-013-0014-z.
27. Martinez-Frias ML, Bermejo E, Rodrigues-Pinilla E, Prieto L. Periconceptional exposure to contraceptive pills and risk for down syndrome. J Perinatol. 2001;21(5):288–92. https://doi.org/10.1038/sj.jp.7210538.
28. Kong YL, Tey HL. Treatment of acne vulgaris during pregnancy and lactation. Drugs. 2013;73(8):779–87. https://doi.org/10.1007/s40265-013-0060-0.
29. James KA, Burkhart CN, Morrell DS. Emerging drugs for acne. Expert Opin Emerg Drugs. 2009;14(4):649–59. https://doi.org/10.1517/14728210903251690.
30. Katsambas A, Dessinioti C. New and emerging treatments in dermatology: acne. Dermatologic Ther. 2008;21(2):86–95. https://doi.org/10.1111/j.1529-8019.2008.00175.x.
31. Dreno B, Blouin E. Acne, pregnant women and zinc salts: a literature review. Ann Dermatol Venereol. 2008;135(1):27–33. https://doi.org/10.1016/j.annder.2007.07.001.
32. Murase JE, Heller MM, Butler DC. Safety of dermatologic medications in pregnancy and lactation: part II. Lactation. J Am Acad Dermatol. 2014;70(3):417.e1–10. https://doi.org/10.1016/j.jaad.2013.09.009.
33. Zeichner JA. Narrowband UV-B phototherapy for the treatment of acne vulgaris during pregnancy. Arch Dermatol. 2011;147(5):537–9. https://doi.org/10.1001/archdermatol.2011.96.
34. Lee KC, Korgavkar K, Dufresne RG, Higgins HW. Safety of cosmetic dermatologic procedures during pregnancy. Dermatol Surg. 2013;39(11):1573–86. https://doi.org/10.1111/dsu.12322.
35. Gerber PA, Buhren BA, Steinhoff M, Homey B. Rosacea: the cytokine and chemokine network. J Investig Dermatol Symp Proc. 2011;15(1):40–7. https://doi.org/10.1038/jidsymp.2011.9.
36. Jarrett R, Gonsalves R, Anstey AV. Differing obstetric outcomes of rosacea fulminans in pregnancy: report of three cases with review of pathogenesis and management. Clin Exp Dermatol. 2010;35(8):888–91. https://doi.org/10.1111/j.1365-2230.2010.03846.x.
37. Jansen T, Plewig G, Kligman AM. Diagnosis and treatment of rosacea fulminans. Dermatology. 1994;188(4):251–4. https://doi.org/10.1159/000247160.
38. de Morais e Silva FA, Bonassi M, Steiner D, da Cunha TV. Rosacea fulminans in pregnancy with ocular perforation. J Dtsch Dermatol Ges. 2011;9(7):542–3. https://doi.org/10.1111/j.1610-0387.2011.07616.x.
39. Spoendlin J, Voegel JJ, Jick SS, Meier CR. A study on the epidemiology of rosacea in the U.K. Br J Dermatol. 2012;167(3):598–605. https://doi.org/10.1111/j.1365-2133.2012.11037.x.
40. Gonzalez-Hinojosa D, Jaime-Villalonga A, Aguilar-Montes G, Lammoglia-Ordiales L. Demodex and rosacea: is there a relationship? Indian J Ophthalmol. 2018;66(1):36–8. https://doi.org/10.4103/ijo.IJO_514_17.
41. Fuentelsaz V, Ara M, Corredera C, Lezcano V, Juberias P, Carapeto FJ. Rosacea fulminans in pregnancy: successful treatment with azithromycin. Clin Exp Dermatol. 2011;36(6):674–6. https://doi.org/10.1111/j.1365-2230.2011.04042.x.

Part III
Skin Cancer and Dermatologic Surgery During Pregnancy

Chapter 7
Skin Cancer in Pregnancy

Jennifer Villasenor-Park

Non-melanoma Skin Cancer

Cutaneous growths or tumors occur during pregnancy and can be benign or malignant. The incidence of both benign and malignant cutaneous lesions will likely increase, as there is a growing trend for women to delay pregnancy [1]. Of these lesions, some are more frequently associated with pregnancy, while the influence of pregnancy on the onset, progression and prognosis of other lesions is still controversial.

Nonmelanoma skin cancer encompasses a variety of cutaneous malignancies that include keratinocyte carcinomas such as basal cell and squamous cell carcinomas, dermatofibromasarcoma protuberans (DFSP), Kaposi sarcoma, Merkel cell carcinoma, and cutaneous lymphoma. While they occur infrequently during pregnancy, they have been described during pregnancy, and their behavior and management during pregnancy will be discussed here.

Keratinocyte carcinomas include basal cell carcinomas and squamous cell carcinomas and are the most common types of skin cancer. These are increasing in incidence, especially within the Medicare population [2, 3]. However, their incidence during pregnancy is unknown. Mucosal involvement by squamous cell carcinoma during pregnancy is well documented and has been reported in the oral mucosa including the tongue and larynx, vulvar region, and cervix [4–6]. There are several case reports of basal cell carcinoma occurring during pregnancy. These reports document unusual and aggressive behavior of basal cell carcinoma occurring during pregnancy, including one case of metastatic basal cell carcinoma, that may not reflect a true effect of pregnancy [7–9]. Interestingly, there are a few reports documenting some association between the use of exogenous hormones and the onset of

J. Villasenor-Park (✉)
Department of Dermatology, University of Pennsylvania, Philadelphia, PA, USA

K. H. Tyler (ed.), *Cutaneous Disorders of Pregnancy*,
https://doi.org/10.1007/978-3-030-49285-4_7

keratinocyte cancer [10–12]. It is thought that photosensitizing agents included in hormonal therapy, particularly estrogen, may increase the risk of nonmelanoma skin cancer [13]. Using a database from the QSkin Sun and Health Study, Olsen et al. studied Caucasian women with no prior history of melanoma or nonmelanoma skin cancer or >5 self-reported ablations for sunspots or skin cancer [14, 15]. After adjusting for age, sun exposure, and phenotypic and lifestyle characteristics, the authors found no significant association between the incidence of basal cell carcinoma or squamous cell carcinoma and the use hormonal therapy or reproductive factors including age at menarche, menopausal status, age at menopause, and parity. They did note a small association between basal cell carcinoma and previous or current use of menopausal hormonal therapy but did not find a dose-response relationship between the two factors. Further longitudinal studies will be helpful to further examine the relationship between exogenous hormones and the onset of nonmelanoma skin cancer.

Merkel cell carcinoma (MCC) is a relatively uncommon, aggressive primary neuroendocrine tumor that typically occurs in elderly patients. It has a high rate of local recurrence and nodal metastasis and low survival rates [16]. It is associated with Merkel cell polyomavirus (MCV), which is thought to play a role in tumorigenesis by tumor-associated antigen expression, insertional mutagenesis, or both [16, 17]. Only four reports of Merkel cell carcinoma during pregnancy are published [18–21], two of which describe the same patient. Chao and Kuppuswami describe the case of a 23-year old woman diagnosed during her second trimester that resulted in metastasis and maternal and fetal demise [18, 20]. Using sensitive Polymerase Chain Reaction (PCR) assay and real-time quantitative PCR, MC polyomavirus could not be detected in fetal autopsy samples from intrauterine fetal deaths despite a high percentage seropositive pregnant women, indicating a lack of evidence for maternal-to-fetal transmission [22]. Given the rare occurrence of Merkel cell carcinoma during pregnancy, it is still unclear whether pregnancy has an effect on the prognosis of Merkel cell carcinoma.

Sebaceous carcinoma, which accounts for less than 1 percent of all cutaneous malignancies, is a rare, aggressive malignant tumor derived from the adnexal epithelium of sebaceous glands. Typically, tumors arise from the adnexa in the periocular region or in extraocular sites. There are only two case reports in the literature of sebaceous carcinoma arising in pregnancy [23, 24]. Both reports described extraocular sebaceous carcinoma arising during pregnancy, and both were treated surgically without complication to the patient or the fetus. Interestingly, one of the patients had an undiagnosed primary lesion present since childhood that grew rapidly during pregnancy, and it is postulated that the immunosuppressive environment that occurs during pregnancy played a role [24].

Kaposi sarcoma (KS) is an angioproliferative disorder that requires infection with human herpes virus 8 (HHV-8) for its development [25]. Although the seroprevalence of HHV-8 is similar between males and females, Kaposi sarcoma is much more common in males, and its growth is repressed in pregnant mice inoculated with KS during early pregnancy when human chorionic gonadotropin (hCG) is elevated [26]. These observations have prompted the hypothesis that female hormones, particularly hCG, have antiproliferative effects on KS. During pregnancy, KS has been observed to spontaneously remit, occur *de novo,* or recur during pregnancy [27]. Additionally, urinary preparations of hCG have been shown to induce apoptosis in KS cells and inhibit KS-associated angiogenesis and matrix metalloprotease activity *in vitro* [28–30]. However, inconsistent effects have been observed in clinical trials using urinary preparations of hCG, which may indicate a contaminating molecule in these preparations that accounts for the anti-proliferative effect observed in other studies [31]. Aggressive and visceral involvement by KS tends to occur in the setting of Human Immunodeficiency Virus (HIV) infection [32–34]. Although vertical transmission is not common, newborns should be evaluated for HHV-8, especially in the setting of HIV infection, as Kaposi sarcoma has been documented in newborns [35, 36].

Dermatofibrosarcoma protuberans is a rare cutaneous sarcoma with an overall incidence of 4.1 per million person-years [37]. Several case reports exist of DFSP occurring *de novo*, growing rapidly, exhibiting more aggressive behavior with fibrosarcomatous change and metastasis during pregnancy suggesting a hormonal role [38–44]. A few case studies have examined the expression of estrogen and progesterone receptors in DFSP, but results have not been consistent, and sample sizes were small [44–46]. Interestingly, Kreicher et al. conducted immunohistochemical studies on archived formalin-fixed, paraffin-embedded tissue from 44 patients with DFSP obtained from a single institution and examined whether there was an association between receptor expression, tumor site, age at diagnosis, sex, race, or disease recurrence [47]. While they did not find a significant association, they did find loss of receptor expression in all recurrent tumors. Based on available published data, women with a history of DFSP who become pregnant should be counseled regarding the risk for recurrence during pregnancy and possible aggressive behavior. Additionally, surgical treatment by either Mohs micrographic surgery or wide local excision with at least 3-cm margins should not be delayed during pregnancy [7].

Mycosis fungoides (MF) or cutaneous T-cell lymphoma (CTCL) is a rare form of non-Hodgkin lymphoma presenting on the skin. MF represents about 4% of all types of non-Hodgkin lymphoma and commonly occurs in older adults with a peak incidence in the sixth to seventh decade; however, MF can occur in the pediatric population [48, 49]. There are only a few case reports describing MF in pregnant patients [50–53]. Amitay-Layish et al. published a single-center retrospective case series of 12 pregnant women with early stage MF (stage I-IB), folliculotropic MF, or parapsoriasis [54]. Most were treated with various modalities prior to pregnancy, ranging from topical steroids to interferon-alpha and isotretinoin. During pregnancy, patients either stopped treatment or were treated with topical steroids and/or phototherapy with narrow-band UVB. There were no women who experienced progression of their disease during or after pregnancy, and most women had normal pregnancies and delivered healthy babies. Another single-center retrospective cohort analysis examined 8 patients, most of whom had early stage disease [55]. Most were in clinical remission at the time of pregnancy, except for one patient who had newly diagnosed stage IIIa CTCL. Most patients experienced an exacerbation of their CTCL shortly after pregnancy, which may be attributed to the relative shift from a Type 1 T helper cell (T_H1) to a Type 2 T helper cell (T_H2) cytokine profile that occurs during pregnancy [54]. Further studies are necessary to determine whether there is an effect of pregnancy on the prognosis of MF.

The occurrence of nonmelanoma skin cancer during pregnancy is relatively rare, and while there are few published data regarding their behavior during pregnancy, appropriate counseling and follow-up are indicated in particular types of nonmelanoma skin cancer. Aggressive cutaneous malignancies, such as dermatofibrosarcoma protuberans and Merkel cell carcinoma, should be treated appropriately during pregnancy and without delay. Additionally, the placenta and the newborn should be examined carefully for possible transmission, especially in the setting of widespread Kaposi sarcoma.

Melanoma in the Pregnant Patient

Pregnancy Associated Changes in Nevi

Hyperpigmentation is one of the most commonly reported skin changes during pregnancy and occurs in up to 90% of women [56, 57]. The exact mechanism of this hyperpigmentation is not clear but has been attributed to hormonal changes, genetics, and UV exposure [58]. Increased levels of beta and alpha melanocyte-stimulating hormone, estrogen, progesterone, and beta-endorphin during pregnancy are thought to lead to melanocyte stimulation and, therefore, hyperpigmentation [57].

Physiologic changes in nevi during pregnancy are more controversial. Historically, changes in nevi have been reported to occur [59]. However, many reports relied on patient observation, and no discernible differences in nevi could be detected when evaluated more objectively [60–62]. Studies assessing changes in the size of nevi during pregnancy did not reveal any significant change. Changes commonly occurred on the abdomen and breasts, which were attributed to the normal stretching of skin that occurs during pregnancy [63–65]. Using in vivo spectrophotometry, Wyon et al. assessed 381 melanocytic nevi on the back and lower legs of pregnant women and compared them with 163 nevi on the backs and lower legs of 21 nulliparous women and found no statistically significant differences in pigmentation [66]. Dermoscopic studies of nevi before, during, and after pregnancy describe transient changes in thickening of pigment network lines, increased brown globules and black dots, and increased vascularity, particularly of nevi on the breasts, abdomen and acral regions. However, these changes regressed 1 year following delivery [67–69]. Increased dermal mitoses and "superficial micronodules of pregnancy," which are clusters of "epithelioid melanocytes with prominent nucleoli, abundant pale eosinophilic cytoplasm, and occasional fine melanosomes," have been reported in histologic studies of nevi biopsied during pregnancy. However, these features were not statistically different when compared to non-pregnant controls [58, 60, 70]. One prospective study of 17 pregnant patients with dysplastic nevus syndrome reported clinical change in 76% of nevi during pregnancy. In addition, these women were two times more likely to have nevi with histologic atypia. One patient was diagnosed with melanoma during pregnancy [71]. Overall, there does not appear to be any significant differences in the clinical, dermoscopic, or histologic appearance of melanocytic nevi during pregnancy in women who do not have dysplastic nevus syndrome. Women with dysplastic nevi should be monitored more closely for changes in their nevi. Importantly, these data suggest that any features suspicious for melanoma should not be attributed to physiologic change and should be treated appropriately.

Pregnancy Associated Melanoma (PAM)

Malignancy during pregnancy is relatively uncommon. However, as more and more women delay pregnancy to their 30s and 40s, a notable increase in the number of malignancies diagnosed during pregnancy has occurred. In the United States, cutaneous melanoma was the fifth most common malignancy amongst new cancer diagnoses in 2019. It represents 5.5% of all new cancer cases in 2019 or 22.2 per 100,000 men and women per year based on cases in 2012 to 2016 [72]. Amongst women between the ages of 20 and 29, melanoma is the second most common malignancy,with an incidence of 6 per 1000 women yearly [73–75]. Nearly one-third of women who are diagnosed with melanoma are of childbearing-age. It is unclear what factor is contributing to these increasing statistics. However, the role of tanning bed use, which is common amongst young women, is likely a contributor to the rise in melanoma amongst this population [76–78]. With these rising statistics, optimal management of patients diagnosed with cutaneous melanoma during pregnancy is critically important.

The prognosis of women diagnosed with pregnancy associated cutaneous melanoma has historically been considered poor. Several anecdotal and case reports starting in the 1950s suggested poor survival, shortened disease-free survival (DFS), and described patients with thicker melanomas [79–81]. Pack et al. reviewed 32 cases of melanoma diagnosed during pregnancy and reported a poor prognosis due to rapid development of metastases [80]. Some reports recommended surgical sterilization due to the perceived poor prognosis of these patients [79]. However, all of these reports had small sample size and lacked controls for stage of disease, depth of melanoma, and the primary site at the time of diagnosis.

The role of hormones in the pathogenesis and progression of melanoma have been the subject of several studies. Estrogens influence several aspects of reproduction, cell growth, development, differentiation, and tumorigenesis, and they exert their effects through both classical estrogen receptors and G protein-coupled estrogen receptors (GPER) [82–85]. Estrogen receptor beta (ERβ) activation is thought to prevent tumor progression, while estrogen receptor alpha (ERα) activation has an opposite effect [86, 87]. The expression of estrogen receptor-alpha in melanoma was first described in 1976; however, estrogen receptor-beta was later found to be the predominant receptor type in melanoma [88–92]. Loss of ERβ expression correlates with increased Breslow depth [91, 93]. Immunohistochemical analyses of melanomas from pregnant and non-pregnant women showed a correlation between GPER/ERβ-positive melanomas and lower Breslow thickness, lower mitotic rate, and higher presence of peritumoral lymphocyte infiltration [94]. Zhou et al. showed more frequent expression of ERβ in pregnant women compared to men; however, there was no difference observed when compared to nonpregnant women, and there was no association between ERβ expression and survival [92]. It is still unclear whether the expression of these receptors and estrogen signaling has a positive or negative impact in the progression of melanoma or survival [95, 96].

The immunologic milieu in the pregnant patient also contributes to the notion of poor prognosis in patients with pregnancy associated melanoma. The immunosuppressive environment necessary for maintaining the fetus during pregnancy has been compared to the environment necessary for cancer and its progression [97, 98]. Specifically, the placental villi, which are in constant contact with maternal blood, do not express Human Leukocyte Antigen (HLA) molecules and therefore do not trigger a maternal T-cell response. The extravillous trophoblast, which are the placental cells that interact with the decidua and myometrium, express only select types of HLA molecules (HLA-C, HLA-E and HLA-G) that do not engage with T cells and mainly engage with receptors on innate immune cells, including natural killer cells and macrophages [99]. Additionally, there is a relative shift from a T_H1-predominant to a T_H2-predominant immune response during pregnancy, leading to suppression of the cytotoxic T-lymphocyte response and a less robust cell-mediated immunity [100]. $CD4^+CD25^+$ regulatory T cells (Tregs) are important for maintaining tolerance to the fetus during pregnancy, and their numbers are notably increased during pregnancy and in cancer [97, 101]. Lastly, uterine natural killer cells (uNKs), which have reduced cytotoxic activity, are present in increased numbers within the maternal-fetal interface of the decidua of the pregnant uterus [97]. To date, there has been no compelling evidence to suggest that the immunologic environment in the pregnant patient predisposes them to or causes the spread of melanoma.

Melanoma Diagnosed during Pregnancy

There is an increase in the number of young women of child-bearing age diagnosed with melanoma. Indeed, the most common malignancy diagnosed during pregnancy is cutaneous melanoma, which represents nearly one-third of all malignancies diagnosed during pregnancy [102]. While reports starting in the 1950s suggested poor prognosis in patients diagnosed with melanoma during pregnancy, more recent reports with larger sample sizes and controls for tumor depth and location using more strict definitions of pregnancy-associated melanoma contradict these original observations. Interestingly, there have been a few studies showing a decreased risk of melanoma in women who are younger at the time of their first child and higher parity compared to women who were older and had fewer than 5 live births, suggesting a protective role of pregnancy in melanoma [103–105].

Additional population-based controlled studies assessing the role of pregnancy in the prognosis of melanoma show no difference in survival. These are summarized in Table 7.1. Lens et al. performed a retrospective cohort study using data from the Swedish National and Regional Registries. A cohort of 185 women diagnosed with melanoma during pregnancy and 5348 women of the same childbearing age diagnosed with melanoma while not pregnant were compared, and no statistically significant difference in overall survival (OS) was found [105]. This group also performed a multivariable Cox regression analysis of the effect of pregnancy subsequent to the diagnosis of melanoma and found no correlation with survival after adjusting for Breslow thickness, tumor site, Clark's level, and age. Tumor thickness and tumor site were better predictors of survival [105].

Using a large California database containing maternal and neonatal discharge records from California between 1991 to 1999 linked to records from the California Cancer Registry, O'Meara et al. found no data to suggest a more advanced stage, thicker tumors, increased metastases to lymph nodes, or decreased survival when comparing women who had pregnancy-associated melanoma (145 antepartum, 4 at delivery, and 263 postpartum) with the control group (2451 women) [106].

Table 7.1 Summary of studies showing no difference in survival in pregnancy associated melanoma

Authors	Study	Population	PAM (N)	Ctrl (N)	Findings	Follow-up
Johannson et al. JAAD 2014	Population-based retrospective cohort	Swedish Cancer and multi-generation registers	1019 (PAM = up to 2 years post-partum)	5838	No difference in cause-specific mortality adjusted for age, tumor location, time since diagnosis	Up to 10 years
Silipo et al. 2006	Single-center retrospective study	Italy	10	30	No difference in outcome and survival	5 years
O'Meara et al. 2005.	Population-based retrospective study	United States (California)	412 (263 first year post-partum; 149 during pregnancy)	2451	No difference in disease, tumor thickness, metastasis to lymph nodes and survival	Up to 10 years
Lens MB et al. J Clin Oncol 2004.	Population-based retrospective cohort	Swedish national and regional registries	185	5348	No difference in survival	Median 11.6 years
Daryanani D et al. Cancer, 2003.	Single center retrospective cohort	Netherlands	46	368	No difference in DFS and OS	Up to 30 years

DFS Disease Free Survival; *OS* Overall Survival; *PAM* Pregnancy Associated Melanoma

Johansson et al. conducted a population-based, retrospective cohort study using the Swedish Cancer and Multi-Generation registers and compared cause-specific mortality in 1019 women with melanoma diagnosed within or less than 2 years postpartum and found no significant difference [107]. Moreover, when their analysis was limited to the 247 women who were diagnosed during pregnancy compared to controls, there was no significant difference in cause-specific mortality.

More recently, Jones et al. performed univariable and multivariable analyses of female patients of reproductive age identified from the prospectively maintained John Wayne Cancer Institute melanoma database. They were compared to a control group of women of similar Breslow thickness, age, stage and ulceration status [108]. No significant differences in disease free survival, melanoma-specific survival, or overall survival were identified on univariable or multivariable analysis for pregnancy-associated melanoma compared to non-pregnant patients.

While many large, controlled studies have been published that do not show an effect on survival in pregnancy-associated melanoma, there have been a few studies published that are discordant with these findings (Table 7.2). However, many of these studies did not report significant differences once they controlled for tumor

Table 7.2 Summary of studies showing increased risk of mortality in pregnancy associated melanoma

Authors	Study	Population	PAM (N)	Control (N)	Findings	Follow-up
Tellez et al. JAAD 2016	Single center retrospective case-control study	Patients at Cleveland Clinic	41; 19 diagnosed during pregnancy	421 remainder of study population	Higher incidence of mortality, recurrence, and metastasis	>2 years follow-up
Byrom Let et al. JEADV 2015	Meta-analysis		10–338		56% increased risk of mortality (based on 4 studies)	5–20 years
Moller et al. 2013	Population-based retrospective study	United Kingdom	306; 29 patients analyzed PAM – 5 years post-partum	3465	2-fold increased risk; risk decreased when adjusted for tumor stage	Up to 11 years
Stensheim et al. JCO 200 g	Population-based retrospective cohort	Norway	247 (diagnosed during pregnancy)	4460	HR 1.52; no diff when adjusted for Breslow thickness and tumor location	Median 11.9 years

PAM Pregnancy Associated Melanoma

thickness and tumor location, and some studies lacked complete data regarding stage of disease. Stenshiem et al. performed a population-based cohort study using data from the Cancer Registry and the Medical Birth Registry of Norway comparing cause-specific survival between pregnant and non-pregnant patients diagnosed with cancer, including breast cancer, cervical cancer, melanoma, lymphoma and leukemia [102]. Amongst those diagnosed with melanoma during pregnancy, the authors found a slightly increased risk of cause-specific death (HR, 1.52; $P = 0.047$). The authors attributed this slightly increased risk to a delay in diagnosis in pregnant patients whose doctors may have interpreted changes in the pigmentation of a mole as a normal physiologic change of pregnancy. When the authors performed a sub-analysis comparing tumor thickness and tumor location amongst pregnant and age-matched, non-pregnant controls, this difference was no longer statistically significant.

Using the national cancer registration and hospital discharge data for women in England from 1998–2007, Moller et al. conducted a population-based retrospective study comparing women diagnosed with melanoma within 5 years post-partum [109]. In their analysis, they found a two-fold increased risk in women who were diagnosed within 1-year post-partum. Within this cohort of patients, 6 of 29 patients were advanced stage (stage III or IV), and 7 patients could not be staged. After adjusting for tumor stage, this association was only slightly attenuated. However, in patients with melanoma diagnosed beyond 1 year but before 5 years postpartum, there was no significant increased risk of cause-specific death. It's unclear whether this observation in women diagnosed within 1 year postpartum is due to a delay in diagnosis during pregnancy, a more aggressive type of melanoma, or a true pregnancy association.

Byrom et al. conducted a meta-analysis of 4 population-based studies utilizing multivariable methods reporting hazard ratios (HR) with confidence intervals (CI) and reported a 56% increased risk of mortality amongst those with pregnancy-associated melanoma [110]. The statistical methods used in this study were reappraised and scrutinized for incomplete data by several authors. Using the same data used by Byrom et al., a repeat analysis did not find any significant differences in mortality amongst women diagnosed with pregnancy-associated melanoma [111, 112].

In 2016, Tellez et al. published a retrospective cohort study using data from a single institution comparing controls to patients diagnosed with melanoma during pregnancy or within 1 year postpartum [113]. In their cohort, 41 patients were included in their analysis, 19 of which were diagnosed during pregnancy. A majority of the patients in this group had advanced stage disease. The authors reported a 20% mortality rate and 5.10 greater odds of death in patients with pregnancy associated melanoma, which is one of the highest reported in the literature. Inconsistent reporting on stage of disease and inappropriate statistical methods have been cited as major flaws in this study [114].

A more recent European observational study published in 2017 used patients selected from the database of the "International Network on Cancer, Infertility, and Pregnancy" (INCIP), which relies on voluntary reporting by doctors who work in specialized hospitals and are affiliated to the INCIP [115]. Sixty patients were included in their analysis, and, amongst this group of patients, there was a high incidence of advanced stage disease. About 50% of patients had regional and metastatic disease (Stage III-IV), which is high compared to the reported incidence of advanced-stage melanoma in young patients (1–5%) [116, 117]. It is likely that the high incidence reported in this study was related to a delay in diagnosis or a referral bias, as these cases were voluntarily reported by physicians affiliated at tertiary care hospitals.

Several studies have assessed the characteristics of melanoma in pregnant patients by evaluating Breslow depth and proliferative activity [81, 102, 105, 106, 118–123]. Two groups did report thicker melanomas in pregnant patients compared to non-pregnant women; however, these studies did not report a difference in survival, and one study found a protective effect on survival [81, 119]. There was also no significant difference in proliferative activity between pregnant and non-pregnant patients diagnosed with melanoma. In a retrospective cohort study conducted at a single institution, pathologists compared melanoma tissue from patients with pregnancy associated melanoma and non-pregnant patients [124]. Tumor proliferation rates were assessed by mitotic count (assessed by the number of dermal mitotic figures/mm^2), phosphohistone H3 staining, and Ki-67 staining. Amongst 50 tissue samples obtained from pregnancy-associated melanoma and 122 tissue samples obtained from non-pregnancy associated melanoma, there were no significant differences in proliferative activity between groups with invasive melanoma. Moreover, no significant association between pregnancy status and Breslow depth, Clark level, or ulceration was noted. Fabian et al. also assessed Breslow thickness and mitotic rate in pregnancy-associated melanoma and compared these rates to non-pregnant women and men and found no significant differences [125].

In summary, most of the data do not support a worse prognosis, increased thickness, or proliferative rate in patients diagnosed with pregnancy associated melanoma.

Melanoma Diagnosed before or after Pregnancy

Several studies have examined whether pregnancy has a negative influence on survival if melanoma is diagnosed before or after pregnancy. Examination of 966 women with melanoma diagnosed before pregnancy compared to 4567 women who did not become pregnant after a melanoma diagnosis showed no difference in survival after controlling for Breslow depth, tumor site, Clark level, and age [105]. Additionally, Mackie et al. examined 85 women who became pregnant after their melanoma diagnosis and compared them to 143 women who did not become pregnant and found no significant difference in overall survival [119].

With regard to the post-partum period, there are a few studies examining the role of pregnancy in the prognosis of melanoma. Johansson et al. examined prognosis in patients with pregnancy associated melanoma up to 5 years postpartum and compared them to controls using data from the Swedish Cancer and Multi-Generation

Registers and found no difference in survival [107]. In a population-based retrospective study conducted in the United Kingdom, Moller et al. did report a two-fold increased risk of mortality in women diagnosed with melanoma within 1 year postpartum [109]. This difference could be attributed to a delay in diagnosis during pregnancy since this difference was no longer significant when comparing women diagnosed more than 1 year postpartum but before 5 years postpartum.

In summary, there does not seem to be a significant impact on survival in patients diagnosed with melanoma before or after pregnancy.

Role of Exogenous Hormones in Pregnancy Associated Melanoma

The expression of estrogen receptors in melanoma is well established [82, 87, 88, 90, 93]. However, the role of exposure to exogenous estrogens and its impact on mortality is not known. There have been several studies examining the role of oral contraceptive pills (OCPs) in the prognosis of melanoma. Early studies reported an increased risk of melanoma in those taking OCPs and suggested a correlation between prolonged use of OCPs and increased risk of developing melanoma [125, 126]. However, these studies did not account for potential confounding factors including a history of sun exposure, and some findings did not reach significance. Larger studies, including two meta-analyses and a pooled analysis of 10 case control studies, showed no correlation between length of use of OCPs, age at first use, or current use and the risk of developing melanoma [127, 128].

The role of HRT in the development of melanoma is less well characterized. One large randomized control trial from the Women's Health Initiative examined the incidence of melanoma in 27,347 postmenopausal women who were randomized to receive either: (1) conjugated equine estrogen plus medroxyprogesterone or placebo (if intact uterus) or (2) estrogen alone or placebo (if had hysterectomy). After 6 years follow-up, there was no detectable difference in the incidence of melanoma between the groups receiving active hormone compared to the placebo group [129].

A recent analysis of 11 studies previously published examined the role of in vitro fertilization (IVF) in melanoma risk compared with the general population [130]. This study also examined the role of different types of IVF in parous or nulliparous women. After analyzing 11 studies that met their criteria, there were no significant patterns indicating an increased risk of melanoma in those patients undergoing IVF compared to the general population. However, in patients who were ever parous either before or after receiving IVF, particularly with use of clomiphene or gonadotropins, there appeared to be an increased risk of melanoma [131–133].

Based on available current evidence, there does not appear to be significant data to suggest any increased risk for developing melanoma in women exposed to exogenous forms of hormones. The current guidelines for the treatment of primary cutaneous melanoma suggest that exogenous hormones may be used in women diagnosed with melanoma [134].

Treatment of Melanoma in the Pregnant Patient

Pregnant patients should be evaluated for any suspicious lesions using the same clinical and dermatoscopic criteria as non-pregnant patients [134]. Pregnant patients diagnosed with melanoma should be managed in the same way as non-pregnant patients. Management by a multidisciplinary team consisting of the obstetrician, neonatologist, oncologist and dermatologist should be the goal in order to adequately evaluate and treat both the mother and the fetus, particularly if the melanoma is at an advanced stage [134–136]. Excisional biopsy of suspicious lesions with 2-mm margins and definitive treatment with appropriate surgical margins based on the depth of the melanoma are current guidelines for the management of melanoma. Surgical treatment in the pregnant patient can be safely performed with appropriate precautions including proper positioning of the patient to avoid aortocaval compression.

For staging and risk assessment, sentinel lymph node biopsy should be considered in patients with melanomas thicker than 0.8 mm and in thinner melanomas with ulceration, as it is helpful in assessing prognosis and guiding treatment [134]. Sentinel lymph node biopsy with lymphoscintigraphy using a radionuclide with a short half-life, such as 99-Techneticum nanocolloid, can be safely performed during pregnancy, as the estimated fetal radiation exposure is less than 0.01 gray (Gy). This is well below the threshold dose of 0.1–0.2 Gy that is associated with fetal malformations. Additionally, no adverse effects on the fetus have been described after sentinel lymph node biopsy during pregnancy [137–139]. As sentinel lymph node biopsy does not influence survival from melanoma, use of this procedure should be considered on a case-by-case basis after thorough discussion of the benefits and risks to the mother and the fetus with a multidisciplinary team.

Treatment of advanced melanoma previously relied on the use of chemotherapy. There are a few reports of successful use of chemotherapy regimens, particularly when used during the second and third trimesters [140–142]. In all cases, full-term delivery should be the goal, if possible, in order to optimize the outcome for the offspring. With the advent of targeted therapy and immunotherapy, the use of these treatments has become standard of care for the treatment of advanced melanoma. However, their use during pregnancy and their effects on the fetus are not well documented. Cytotoxic T-lymphocyte-associated protein 4 (CTLA-4) blockade with ipilimumab, an Immunoglobulin G1 (IgG1) antibody, can cross the placenta, and animal studies in monkeys show in an increased rate of miscarriage, still births, premature births, malformation of the urogenital tract, and neonatal death [143]. There are only a few case reports of successful delivery of a healthy baby following in utero exposure to ipilumumab during pregnancy [144, 145]. The Programmed cell death-1 (PD-1) inhibitors such as nivolumab and pembrolizumab, both Immunoglobulin G4 (IgG4) antibodies, also cross the placenta with the highest risk for transplacental transfer during the third trimester. Use of PD-1 inhibitors led to fetal loss in pregnant mice [143]. There are few reports of PD-1 inhibitor use during pregnancy in humans. Menzer et al. describe the use of a combination of ipilimumab and nivolumab in a stage IV melanoma patient during pregnancy with the resultant delivery of a healthy baby with no evidence of melanoma [145].

BRAF inhibitors, specifically vemurafenib, have not been studied for their use in pregnancy; however, only a few case studies have been reported. The earliest case reported for use of vemurafenib during pregnancy was in 2013 in a 37 year old woman with metastatic melanoma [146]. She was given vemurafenib during her second trimester of pregnancy at the 25th week with the hope of prolonging the duration of gestation until week 34. However, the growth of the fetus rapidly declined, and the patient underwent caesarian section during 30th week of gestation due to fetal distress. Since restriction of growth was already observed during the 24th week of gestation before the initiation of vemurafenib therapy, it is unclear whether the continued decline in growth observed after the initiation of vemurafenib was due to maternal illness or a toxic effect from vemurafenib. There were no fetal malformations reported. Another case report describes the successful treatment of a 25 year-old woman, gravida 1, with a history of stage IIA melanoma diagnosed and treated with wide local excision and a negative sentinel lymph node biopsy 5 years prior to presentation [147]. She was diagnosed with Stage IV metastatic melanoma with metastasis to the lungs and treated with vemurafenib starting at 25 weeks of gestation. She delivered a female infant with a birth weight in the 67th percentile and APGAR scores of 9 and 9 at 34 weeks of gestation. The neonatal course was complicated by paroxysmal supraventricular tachycardia requiring admission to the neonatal intensive care unit (NICU). No congenital malformations or melanoma were reported in the infant. Finally, de Haan et al. describe a case of a 30 year old woman with widely metastatic melanoma and a twin pregnancy who was treated with vemurafenib starting at week 22 of gestation and developed toxic epidermal necrolysis (TEN) 12 days after commencing treatment with vemurafenib [148]. The patient delivered at 26 weeks of gestation while under sedation. After a prolonged stay at the NICU, the twins appeared to be developing normally.

Previous studies on the effect of chemotherapy during pregnancy have shown that chemotherapy after the first trimester is unlikely to have long-term effects on the development of the exposed offspring, while prematurity negatively impacts offspring developmental outcomes [141, 142]. However, in cases where conventional chemotherapy fails to improve prognosis, the use of targeted therapy or immunotherapy are increasingly being considered.

Family Planning Following Melanoma Diagnosis

There is no convincing evidence to suggest a worst prognosis for women who become pregnant following the diagnosis and treatment of melanoma [105, 119]. For women diagnosed and treated for early stage melanoma (melanoma in situ or stage I), there is little risk for metastasis. Therefore, a prolonged waiting period prior to subsequent pregnancy is not recommended [134]. For women with advanced stage melanoma, the recommendations for subsequent pregnancies should be determined on a case-by-case basis, and factors such as the thickness and stage of melanoma, age, and fertility of the mother should all be considered. Specifically, women with more advanced stage melanoma, stage II or higher, should consider a 2 to 3 year delay prior to subsequent pregnancies due to the relatively high risk for recurrences that can develop during this time. This recommendation is based on possible complications that can arise during systemic treatment of advanced melanoma during pregnancy. In addition, melanoma is the most common malignancy to metastasize to the placenta and the fetus during pregnancy [149, 150]. Therefore, in patients with metastatic melanoma during pregnancy, careful examination of the placenta is important to rule out placental involvement. With placental involvement, the risk of metastasis to the fetus is thought to be about 22% [151].

Summary

Women diagnosed with melanoma before, during, or after pregnancy do not have a worse prognosis than non-pregnant patients. While hyperpigmentation of the skin occurs during pregnancy, any suspicious melanocytic lesion should be biopsied, which can be done safely during pregnancy. Surgical treatment of melanoma during pregnancy should follow appropriate guidelines and should not be delayed. In advanced stage patients, treatment by a multidisciplinary team composed of obstetricians, oncologists, neonatologists, and dermatologists is important to ensure optimal care and appropriate consideration of risks of therapeutic options for both the mother and the fetus.

References

1. Matthews TJ, Hamilton BE. Delayed childbearing: more women are having their first child later in life. NCHS Data Brief. 2009;21:1–8.
2. Christenson LJ, Borrowman TA, Vachon CM, Tollefson MM, Otley CC, Weaver AL, Roenigk RK. Incidence of basal cell and squamous cell carcinomas in a population younger than 40 years. JAMA. 2005;294(6):681–90. https://doi.org/10.1001/jama.294.6.681.
3. Rogers HW, Weinstock MA, Feldman SR, Coldiron BM. Incidence estimate of nonmelanoma skin Cancer (keratinocyte carcinomas) in the U.S. population, 2012. JAMA Dermatol. 2015;151(10):1081–6. https://doi.org/10.1001/jamadermatol.2015.1187.
4. Pugi J, Levin M, Gupta M. Supraglottic p16+ squamous cell carcinoma during pregnancy: a case report and review of the literature. J Otolaryngol Head Neck Surg. 2019;48(1):47. https://doi.org/10.1186/s40463-019-0378-z.
5. Murphy J, Berman DR, Edwards SP, Prisciandaro J, Eisbruch A, Ward BB. Squamous cell carcinoma of the tongue during pregnancy: a case report and review of the literature. J Oral Maxillofac Surg. 2016;74(12):2557–66. https://doi.org/10.1016/j.joms.2016.06.173.
6. Karrberg C, Radberg T, Holmberg E, Norstrom A. Support for down-staging of pregnancy-associated cervical cancer. Acta Obstet Gynecol Scand. 2015;94(6):654–9. https://doi.org/10.1111/aogs.12645.
7. Walker JL, Wang AR, Kroumpouzos G, Weinstock MA. Cutaneous tumors in pregnancy. Clin Dermatol. 2016;34(3):359–67. https://doi.org/10.1016/j.clindermatol.2016.02.008.

8. Fisher GH, Bangash SJ, Mones J, Geronemus RG. Rapid growth of basal cell carcinoma in a multigestational pregnancy. Dermatol Surg. 2006;32(11):1418–20. https://doi.org/10.1111/j.1524-4725.2006.32316.x.
9. Sass U, Theunis A, Noel JC, Andre J, Song M. Multiple HPV-positive basal cell carcinomas on the abdomen in a young pregnant woman. Dermatology. 2002;204(4):362–4. https://doi.org/10.1159/000063386.
10. Birch-Johansen F, Jensen A, Olesen AB, Christensen J, Tjonneland A, Kjaer SK. Does hormone replacement therapy and use of oral contraceptives increase the risk of non-melanoma skin cancer? Cancer Causes Control. 2012;23(2):379–88. https://doi.org/10.1007/s10552-011-9887-4.
11. Cahoon EK, Kitahara CM, Ntowe E, Bowen EM, Doody MM, Alexander BH, Lee T, Little MP, Linet MS, Freedman DM. Female estrogen-related factors and incidence of basal cell carcinoma in a Nationwide US cohort. J Clin Oncol. 2015;33(34):4058–65. https://doi.org/10.1200/JCO.2015.62.0625.
12. Kuklinski LF, Zens MS, Perry AE, Gossai A, Nelson HH, Karagas MR. Sex hormones and the risk of keratinocyte cancers among women in the United States: a population-based case-control study. Int J Cancer. 2016;139(2):300–9. https://doi.org/10.1002/ijc.30072.
13. Robinson SN, Zens MS, Perry AE, Spencer SK, Duell EJ, Karagas MR. Photosensitizing agents and the risk of non-melanoma skin cancer: a population-based case-control study. J Invest Dermatol. 2013;133(8):1950–5. https://doi.org/10.1038/jid.2013.33.
14. Olsen CM, Green AC, Neale RE, Webb PM, Cicero RA, Jackman LM, O'Brien SM, Perry SL, Ranieri BA, Whiteman DC, Study QS. Cohort profile: the QSkin sun and health study. Int J Epidemiol. 2012;41(4):929–929i. https://doi.org/10.1093/ije/dys107.
15. Olsen CM, Pandeya N, Thompson BS, Dusingize JC, Subramaniam P, Nagle CM, Green AC, Neale RE, Webb PM, Whiteman DC. Hormonal and reproductive factors and incidence of basal cell carcinoma and squamous cell carcinoma in a large, prospective cohort. J Am Acad Dermatol. 2018;78(3):615–618.e612. https://doi.org/10.1016/j.jaad.2017.09.033.
16. Coggshall K, Tello TL, North JP, Yu SS. Merkel cell carcinoma: an update and review: pathogenesis, diagnosis, and staging. J Am Acad Dermatol. 2018;78(3):433–42. https://doi.org/10.1016/j.jaad.2017.12.001.
17. Feng H, Shuda M, Chang Y, Moore PS. Clonal integration of a Polyomavirus in human Merkel cell carcinoma. Science. 2008;319(5866):1096–100. https://doi.org/10.1126/science.1152586.
18. Chao TC, Park JM, Rhee H, Greager JA. Merkel cell tumor of the back detected during pregnancy. Plast Reconstr Surg. 1990;86(2):347–51. https://doi.org/10.1097/00006534-199008000-00028.
19. Kukko H, Vuola J, Suominen S, Koljonen V. Merkel cell carcinoma in a young pregnant woman. J Plast Reconstruct Aesthet Surg. 2008;61(12):1530–3. https://doi.org/10.1016/j.bjps.2007.06.016.
20. Kuppuswami N, Sivarajan KM, Hussein L, Ray VH, Freese UE. Merkel cell tumor in pregnancy. A case report. J Reprod Med. 1991;36(8):613–5.
21. Paterson C, Musselman L, Chorneyko K, Reid S, Rawlinson J. Merkel cell (neuroendocrine) carcinoma of the Anal Canal. Dis Colon Rectum. 2003;46(5):676–8. https://doi.org/10.1007/s10350-004-6630-1.
22. Sadeghi M, Riipinen A, Vaisanen E, Chen T, Kantola K, Surcel HM, Karikoski R, Taskinen H, Soderlund-Venermo M, Hedman K. Newly discovered KI, WU, and Merkel cell polyomaviruses: no evidence of mother-to-fetus transmission. Virol J. 2010;7:251. https://doi.org/10.1186/1743-422x-7-251.
23. Crandall M, Satter EK, Hurt M. Extraocular sebaceous carcinoma arising in a nevus sebaceous during pregnancy. J Am Acad Dermatol. 2012;67(3):e111–3. https://doi.org/10.1016/j.jaad.2011.09.019.
24. Ghosh SK, Bandyopadhyay D, Gupta S, Chatterjee G, Ghosh A. Rapidly growing extraocular sebaceous carcinoma occurring during pregnancy: a case report. Dermatol Online J. 2008;14(8):8.

25. Gao SJ, Kingsley L, Hoover DR, Spira TJ, Rinaldo CR, Saah A, Phair J, Detels R, Parry P, Chang Y, Moore PS. Seroconversion to antibodies against Kaposi's sarcoma-associated herpesvirus-related latent nuclear antigens before the development of Kaposi's sarcoma. N Engl J Med. 1996;335(4):233–41. https://doi.org/10.1056/nejm199607253350403.
26. Lunardi-Iskandar Y, Bryant JL, Zeman RA, Lam VH, Samaniego F, Besnier JM, Hermans P, Thierry AR, Gill P, Gallo RC. Tumorigenesis and metastasis of neoplastic Kaposi's sarcoma cell line in immunodeficient mice blocked by a human pregnancy hormone. Nature. 1995;375(6526):64–8. https://doi.org/10.1038/375064a0.
27. Brunet-Possenti F, Pages C, Rouzier R, Dupin N, Bagot M, Lebbe C. Kaposi's sarcoma and pregnancy: case report and literature review. Dermatology. 2013;226(4):311–4. https://doi.org/10.1159/000349987.
28. Masood R, McGarvey ME, Zheng T, Cai J, Arora N, Smith DL, Sloane N, Gill PS. Antineoplastic urinary protein inhibits Kaposi's sarcoma and angiogenesis in vitro and in vivo. Blood. 1999;93(3):1038–44.
29. Pfeffer U, Bisacchi D, Morini M, Benelli R, Minghelli S, Vacca A, Noonan DM, Albini A. Human chorionic gonadotropin inhibits Kaposi's sarcoma associated angiogenesis, matrix metalloprotease activity, and tumor growth. Endocrinology. 2002;143(8):3114–21. https://doi.org/10.1210/endo.143.8.8945.
30. Samaniego F, Bryant JL, Liu N, Karp JE, Sabichi AL, Thierry A, Lunardi-Iskandar Y, Gallo RC. Induction of programmed cell death in Kaposi's sarcoma cells by preparations of human chorionic gonadotropin. J Natl Cancer Inst. 1999;91(2):135–43. https://doi.org/10.1093/jnci/91.2.135.
31. Bisacchi D, Noonan DM, Carlone S, Albini A, Pfeffer U. Kaposi's sarcoma and human chorionic gonadotropin: mechanisms, moieties and mysteries. Biol Chem. 2002;383(9):1315–20. https://doi.org/10.1515/bc.2002.149.
32. Mian DB, Itoua C, Angoi V, Gbary E, Nguessan KL, Iloki H, Boni S. Late diagnosis of positive HIV serology in pregnancy incidentally discovered by the widespread appearance of Kaposi's sarcoma. Clin Exp Obstet Gynecol. 2015;42(3):378–80.
33. Bryant AE, Genc M, Hurtado RM, Chen KT. Pulmonary Kaposi's sarcoma in pregnancy. Am J Perinatol. 2004;21(6):355–63. https://doi.org/10.1055/s-2004-831880.
34. Rawlinson KF, Zubrow AB, Harris MA, Jackson UC, Chao S. Disseminated Kaposi's sarcoma in pregnancy: a manifestation of acquired immune deficiency syndrome. Obstet Gynecol. 1984;63(3 Suppl):2s–6s.
35. Gutierrez-Ortega P, Hierro-Orozco S, Sanchez-Cisneros R, Montano LF. Kaposi's sarcoma in a 6-day-old infant with human immunodeficiency virus. Arch Dermatol. 1989;125(3):432–3.
36. McCarty KA, Bungu Z. Kaposi's sarcoma in a two week old infant born to a mother with Kaposi's sarcoma/AIDS. Cent Afr J Med. 1995;41(10):330–1.
37. Kreicher KL, Kurlander DE, Gittleman HR, Barnholtz-Sloan JS, Bordeaux JS. Incidence and survival of primary Dermatofibrosarcoma Protuberans in the United States. Dermatol Surg. 2016;42:S24–31. https://doi.org/10.1097/dss.0000000000000300.
38. Anderson KA, Vidimos AT. Two primary dermatofibrosarcoma protuberans associated with different pregnancies in a single patient. Dermatol Surg. 2012;38(11):1876–8. https://doi.org/10.1111/j.1524-4725.2012.02519.x.
39. Bigby SM, Oei P, Lambie NK, Symmans PJ. Dermatofibrosarcoma protuberans: report of a case with a variant ring chromosome and metastases following pregnancy. J Cutan Pathol. 2006;33(5):383–8. https://doi.org/10.1111/j.0303-6987.2006.00404.x.
40. Byekova Y, Marrazzo G, Thorpe R, Susa J, Taylor S. Fibrosarcomatous transformation of a Dermatofibrosarcoma Protuberans during pregnancy. Dermatol Surg. 2015;41(9):1077–9. https://doi.org/10.1097/dss.0000000000000411.
41. Cakir B, Misirlioglu A, Gideroglu K, Akoz T. Giant fibrosarcoma arising in dermatofibrosarcoma protuberans on the scalp during pregnancy. Dermatol Surg. 2003;29(3):297–9. https://doi.org/10.1046/j.1524-4725.2003.29066.x.

42. Har-Shai Y, Govrin-Yehudain J, Ullmann Y, Kerner H, Cohen HI, Lichtig C, Bergman R, Cohen A, Kuten A, Friedman-Birnbaum R, et al. Dermatofibrosarcoma protuberans appearing during pregnancy. Ann Plast Surg. 1993;31(1):91–3.
43. Morrison AE, Lang PG. Case of rapidly enlarging Dermatofibrosarcoma protuberans during pregnancy followed by metastasis in the absence of local recurrence. Dermatol Surg. 2006;32(1):125–7. https://doi.org/10.1111/1524-4725.2006.32020.
44. Parlette LE, Smith CK, Germain LM, Rolfe CA, Skelton H. Accelerated growth of dermatofibrosarcoma protuberans during pregnancy. J Am Acad Dermatol. 1999;41(5 Pt 1):778–83. https://doi.org/10.1016/s0190-9622(99)70023-x.
45. Ghorbani RP, Malpica A, Ayala AG. Dermatofibrosarcoma protuberans of the vulva: clinicopathologic and immunohistochemical analysis of four cases, one with fibrosarcomatous change, and review of the literature. Int J Gynecol Pathol. 1999;18(4):366–73.
46. Schwartz BM, Kuo DYS, Goldberg GL. Dermatofibrosarcoma Protuberans of the vulva: a rare tumor presenting during pregnancy in a teenager. J Low Genit Tract Dis. 1999;3(2):139–42. https://doi.org/10.1046/j.1526-0976.1999.08101.x.
47. Kreicher KL, Honda KS, Kurlander DE, Bordeaux JS. Hormone receptor expression in patients with dermatofibrosarcoma protuberans. J Am Acad Dermatol. 2016;75(6):1205–9. https://doi.org/10.1016/j.jaad.2016.07.011.
48. Crowley JJ, Nikko A, Varghese A, Hoppe RT, Kim YH. Mycosis fungoides in young patients: clinical characteristics and outcome. J Am Acad Dermatol. 1998;38(5 Pt 1):696–701. https://doi.org/10.1016/s0190-9622(98)70198-7.
49. Ferenczi K, Makkar HS. Cutaneous lymphoma: kids are not just little people. Clin Dermatol. 2016;34(6):749–59. https://doi.org/10.1016/j.clindermatol.2016.07.010.
50. Castelo-Branco C, Torne A, Cararach V, Iglesias X. Mycosis fungoides and pregnancy. Oncol Rep. 2001;8(1):197–9. https://doi.org/10.3892/or.8.1.197.
51. Echols KT, Gilles JM, Diro M. Mycosis fungoides in pregnancy: remission after treatment with alpha-interferon in a case refractory to conventional therapy: a case report. J Matern Fetal Med. 2001;10(1):68–70. https://doi.org/10.1080/714052707.
52. Naeini FF, Najafian J, Nilforoushzadeh M. CD30+ large cell transformation of mycosis Fungoides during pregnancy. Indian J Dermatol. 2013;58(2):160. https://doi.org/10.4103/0019-5154.108090.
53. Dalton SR, Hicks M, Shabanowitz R, Elston DM. Ethical dilemmas in the management of tumor-stage mycosis fungoides in a pregnant patient. J Am Acad Dermatol. 2012;66(4):661–3. https://doi.org/10.1016/j.jaad.2011.11.952.
54. Amitay-Layish I, David M, Kafri B, Barzilai A, Feinmesser M, Hodak E. Early-stage mycosis fungoides, parapsoriasis en plaque, and pregnancy. Int J Dermatol. 2007;46(2):160–5. https://doi.org/10.1111/j.1365-4632.2006.02963.x.
55. Fatemi Naeini F, Abtahi-Naeini B, Najafian J, Saffaei A, Pourazizi M. Correlation between mycosis fungoides and pregnancy. Saudi Med J. 2016;37(9):968–72. https://doi.org/10.15537/smj.2016.9.15838.
56. Motosko CC, Bieber AK, Pomeranz MK, Stein JA, Martires KJ. Physiologic changes of pregnancy: a review of the literature. International Journal of Women's Dermatology. 2017;3(4):219–24. https://doi.org/10.1016/j.ijwd.2017.09.003.
57. Tyler KH. Physiological skin changes during pregnancy. Clin Obstet Gynecol. 2015;58(1):119–24. https://doi.org/10.1097/GRF.0000000000000077.
58. Bieber AK, Martires KJ, Driscoll MS, Grant-Kels JM, Pomeranz MK, Stein JA. Nevi and pregnancy. J Am Acad Dermatol. 2016;75(4):661–6. https://doi.org/10.1016/j.jaad.2016.01.060.
59. Winton GB, Lewis CW. Dermatoses of pregnancy. J Am Acad Dermatol. 1982;6(6):977–98. https://doi.org/10.1016/s0190-9622(82)70083-0.
60. Foucar E, Bentley TJ, Laube DW, Rosai J. A histopathologic evaluation of nevocellular nevi in pregnancy. Arch Dermatol. 1985;121(3):350–4.

61. Grin CM, Rojas AI, Grant-Kels JM. Does pregnancy alter melanocytic nevi? J Cutan Pathol. 2001;28(8):389–92. https://doi.org/10.1034/j.1600-0560.2001.028008389.x.
62. Muzaffar F, Hussain I, Haroon TS. Physiologic skin changes during pregnancy: a study of 140 cases. Int J Dermatol. 1998;37(6):429–31. https://doi.org/10.1046/j.1365-4362.1998.00281.x.
63. Akturk AS, Bilen N, Bayramgurler D, Demirsoy EO, Erdogan S, Kiran R. Dermoscopy is a suitable method for the observation of the pregnancy-related changes in melanocytic nevi. J Eur Acad Dermatol Venereol. 2007;21(8):1086–90. https://doi.org/10.1111/j.1468-3083.2007.02204.x.
64. Pennoyer JW, Grin CM, Driscoll MS, Dry SM, Walsh SJ, Gelineau JP, Grant-Kels JM. Changes in size of melanocytic nevi during pregnancy. J Am Acad Dermatol. 1997;36(3 Pt 1):378–82. https://doi.org/10.1016/s0190-9622(97)80212-5.
65. Strumia R. Digital epiluminescence microscopy in nevi during pregnancy. Dermatology. 2002;205(2):186–7. https://doi.org/10.1159/000063901.
66. Wyon Y, Synnerstad I, Fredrikson M, Rosdahl I. Spectrophotometric analysis of melanocytic naevi during pregnancy. Acta Derm Venereol. 2007;87(3):231–7. https://doi.org/10.2340/00015555-0227.
67. Gunduz K, Koltan S, Sahin MT, Filiz E. Analysis of melanocytic naevi by dermoscopy during pregnancy. J Eur Acad Dermatol Venereol. 2003;17(3):349–51. https://doi.org/10.1046/j.1468-3083.2003.00792_2.x.
68. Nachbar F, Stolz W, Merkle T, Cognetta AB, Vogt T, Landthaler M, Bilek P, Braun-Falco O, Plewig G. The ABCD rule of dermatoscopy. High prospective value in the diagnosis of doubtful melanocytic skin lesions. J Am Acad Dermatol. 1994;30(4):551–9. https://doi.org/10.1016/s0190-9622(94)70061-3.
69. Zampino MR, Corazza M, Costantino D, Mollica G, Virgili A. Are melanocytic nevi influenced by pregnancy? A dermoscopic evaluation. Dermatol Surg. 2006;32(12):1497–504. https://doi.org/10.1111/j.1524-4725.2006.32362.x.
70. Chan MP, Chan MM, Tahan SR. Melanocytic nevi in pregnancy: histologic features and Ki-67 proliferation index. J Cutan Pathol. 2010;37(8):843–51. https://doi.org/10.1111/j.1600-0560.2009.01491.x.
71. Ellis DL. Pregnancy and sex steroid hormone effects on nevi of patients with the dysplastic nevus syndrome. J Am Acad Dermatol. 1991;25(3):467–82. https://doi.org/10.1016/0190-9622(91)70227-S.
72. Howlader N NA, Krapcho M, Miller D, Brest A, Yu M, Ruhl J, Tatalovich Z, Mariotto A, Lewis DR, Chen HS, Feuer EJ, Cronin KA (2019)SEER Cancer statistics review, 1975-2016. https://seer.cancer.gov/statfacts/html/melan.html. Accessed 21 Dec 2019.
73. Watson M, Geller AC, Tucker MA, Guy GP, Weinstock MA. Melanoma burden and recent trends among non-Hispanic whites aged 15–49 years, United States. Prevent Med. 2016;91:294–8. https://doi.org/10.1016/j.ypmed.2016.08.032.
74. Lee YY, Roberts CL, Dobbins T, Stavrou E, Black K, Morris J, Young J. Incidence and outcomes of pregnancy-associated cancer in Australia, 1994-2008: a population-based linkage study. BJOG. 2012;119(13):1572–82. https://doi.org/10.1111/j.1471-0528.2012.03475.x.
75. Pereg D, Koren G, Lishner M. Cancer in pregnancy: gaps, challenges and solutions. Cancer Treat Rev. 2008;34(4):302–12. https://doi.org/10.1016/j.ctrv.2008.01.002.
76. Ghiasvand R, Rueegg CS, Weiderpass E, Green AC, Lund E, Veierod MB. Indoor tanning and melanoma risk: long-term evidence from a prospective population-based cohort study. Am J Epidemiol. 2017;185(3):147–56. https://doi.org/10.1093/aje/kww148.
77. Lazovich D, Isaksson Vogel R, Weinstock MA, Nelson HH, Ahmed RL, Berwick M. Association between indoor tanning and melanoma in younger men and women. JAMA Dermatol. 2016;152(3):268–75. https://doi.org/10.1001/jamadermatol.2015.2938.
78. Ghiasvand R, Robsahm TE, Green AC, Rueegg CS, Weiderpass E, Lund E, Veierod MB. Association of Phenotypic Characteristics and UV radiation exposure with risk of melanoma on different body sites. JAMA Dermatol. 2019;155(1):39–49. https://doi.org/10.1001/jamadermatol.2018.3964.

79. Byrd BF Jr, Mc GW. The effect of pregnancy on the clinical course of malignant melanoma. South Med J. 1954;47(3):196–200. https://doi.org/10.1097/00007611-195403000-00002.
80. Pack GT, Scharnagel IM. The prognosis for malignant melanoma in the pregnant woman. Cancer. 1951;4(2):324–34. https://doi.org/10.1002/1097-0142(195103)4:2<324::aid-cncr2820040218>3.0.co;2-g.
81. Travers RL, Sober AJ, Berwick M, Mihm MC Jr, Barnhill RL, Duncan LM. Increased thickness of pregnancy-associated melanoma. Br J Dermatol. 1995;132(6):876–83. https://doi.org/10.1111/j.1365-2133.1995.tb16942.x.
82. Hewitt SC, Korach KS. Estrogen receptors: new directions in the new millennium. Endocr Rev. 2018;39(5):664–75. https://doi.org/10.1210/er.2018-00087.
83. Ascenzi P, Bocedi A, Marino M. Structure-function relationship of estrogen receptor alpha and beta: impact on human health. Mol Asp Med. 2006;27(4):299–402. https://doi.org/10.1016/j.mam.2006.07.001.
84. Filardo EJ, Quinn JA, Bland KI, Frackelton AR Jr. Estrogen-induced activation of Erk-1 and Erk-2 requires the G protein-coupled receptor homolog, GPR30, and occurs via trans-activation of the epidermal growth factor receptor through release of HB-EGF. Mol Endocrinol. 2000;14(10):1649–60. https://doi.org/10.1210/mend.14.10.0532.
85. Filardo EJ, Quinn JA, Frackelton AR Jr, Bland KI. Estrogen action via the G protein-coupled receptor, GPR30: stimulation of adenylyl cyclase and cAMP-mediated attenuation of the epidermal growth factor receptor-to-MAPK signaling axis. Mol Endocrinol. 2002;16(1):70–84. https://doi.org/10.1210/mend.16.1.0758.
86. Bardin A, Boulle N, Lazennec G, Vignon F, Pujol P. Loss of ERbeta expression as a common step in estrogen-dependent tumor progression. Endocr Relat Cancer. 2004;11(3):537–51. https://doi.org/10.1677/erc.1.00800.
87. Helguero LA, Faulds MH, Gustafsson JA, Haldosen LA. Estrogen receptors alfa (ERalpha) and beta (ERbeta) differentially regulate proliferation and apoptosis of the normal murine mammary epithelial cell line HC11. Oncogene. 2005;24(44):6605–16. https://doi.org/10.1038/sj.onc.1208807.
88. Fisher RI, Neifeld JP, Lippman ME. Oestrogen receptors in human malignant melanoma. Lancet. 1976;2(7981):337–9. https://doi.org/10.1016/s0140-6736(76)92592-7.
89. H-J GRILL, BENES P, MANZ B, MORSCHES B, KORTING GW, POLLOW K. Steroid hormone receptor analysis in human melanoma and non-malignant human skin. Br J Dermatol. 1982;107(s23):64–5. https://doi.org/10.1111/j.1365-2133.1982.tb01035.x.
90. OHATA C, TADOKORO T, ITAMI S. Expression of estrogen receptor β in normal skin, melanocytic nevi and malignant melanomas. J Dermatol. 2008;35(4):215–21. https://doi.org/10.1111/j.1346-8138.2008.00447.x.
91. Schmidt AN, Nanney LB, Boyd AS, King LE Jr, Ellis DL. Oestrogen receptor-beta expression in melanocytic lesions. Exp Dermatol. 2006;15(12):971–80. https://doi.org/10.1111/j.1600-0625.2006.00502.x.
92. Zhou JH, Kim KB, Myers JN, Fox PS, Ning J, Bassett RL, Hasanein H, Prieto VG. Immunohistochemical expression of hormone receptors in melanoma of pregnant women, nonpregnant women, and men. Am J Dermatopathol. 2014;36(1):74–9. https://doi.org/10.1097/DAD.0b013e3182914c64.
93. de Giorgi V, Gori A, Gandini S, Papi F, Grazzini M, Rossari S, Simoni A, Maio V, Massi D. Oestrogen receptor beta and melanoma: a comparative study. Br J Dermatol. 2013;168(3):513–9. https://doi.org/10.1111/bjd.12056.
94. Fábián M, Rencz F, Krenács T, Brodszky V, Hársing J, Németh K, Balogh P, Kárpáti S. Expression of G protein-coupled oestrogen receptor in melanoma and in pregnancy-associated melanoma. J Eur Acad Dermatol Venereol. 2017;31(9):1453–61. https://doi.org/10.1111/jdv.14304.
95. Natale CA, Li J, Zhang J, Dahal A, Dentchev T, Stanger BZ, Ridky TW. Activation of G protein-coupled estrogen receptor signaling inhibits melanoma and improves response to immune checkpoint blockade. eLife. 2018;7:e31770. https://doi.org/10.7554/eLife.31770.

96. Tian W, Pang W, Ge Y, He X, Wang D, Li X, Hou H, Zhou D, Feng S, Chen Z, Yang Y. Hepatocyte-generated 27-hydroxycholesterol promotes the growth of melanoma by activation of estrogen receptor alpha. J Cell Biochem. 2018;119(3):2929–38. https://doi.org/10.1002/jcb.26498.
97. Holtan SG, Creedon DJ, Haluska P, Markovic SN. Cancer and pregnancy: parallels in growth, invasion, and immune modulation and implications for cancer therapeutic agents. Mayo Clin Proc. 2009;84(11):985–1000. https://doi.org/10.1016/S0025-6196(11)60669-1.
98. Flint TR, Jones JO, Ferrer M, Colucci F, Janowitz T. A comparative analysis of immune privilege in pregnancy and cancer in the context of checkpoint blockade immunotherapy. Semin Oncol. 2018;45(3):170–5. https://doi.org/10.1053/j.seminoncol.2018.03.005.
99. Apps R, Murphy SP, Fernando R, Gardner L, Ahad T, Moffett A. Human leucocyte antigen (HLA) expression of primary trophoblast cells and placental cell lines, determined using single antigen beads to characterize allotype specificities of anti-HLA antibodies. Immunology. 2009;127(1):26–39. https://doi.org/10.1111/j.1365-2567.2008.03019.x.
100. Pazos M, Sperling RS, Moran TM, Kraus TA. The influence of pregnancy on systemic immunity. Immunol Res. 2012;54(1–3):254–61. https://doi.org/10.1007/s12026-012-8303-9.
101. Leber A, Teles A, Zenclussen AC. Regulatory T cells and their role in pregnancy. Am J Reprod Immunol. 2010;63(6):445–59. https://doi.org/10.1111/j.1600-0897.2010.00821.x.
102. Stensheim H, Moller B, van Dijk T, Fossa SD. Cause-specific survival for women diagnosed with cancer during pregnancy or lactation: a registry-based cohort study. J Clin Oncol. 2009;27(1):45–51. https://doi.org/10.1200/JCO.2008.17.4110.
103. Gandini S, Iodice S, Koomen E, Di Pietro A, Sera F, Caini S. Hormonal and reproductive factors in relation to melanoma in women: current review and meta-analysis. Eur J Cancer. 2011;47(17):2607–17. https://doi.org/10.1016/j.ejca.2011.04.023.
104. Karagas MR, Zens MS, Stukel TA, Swerdlow AJ, Rosso S, Osterlind A, Mack T, Kirkpatrick C, Holly EA, Green A, Gallagher R, Elwood JM, Armstrong BK. Pregnancy history and incidence of melanoma in women: a pooled analysis. Cancer Causes Control. 2006;17(1):11–9. https://doi.org/10.1007/s10552-005-0281-y.
105. Lens MB, Rosdahl I, Ahlbom A, Farahmand BY, Synnerstad I, Boeryd B, Newton Bishop JA. Effect of pregnancy on survival in women with cutaneous malignant melanoma. J Clin Oncol. 2004;22(21):4369–75. https://doi.org/10.1200/JCO.2004.02.096.
106. O'Meara AT, Cress R, Xing G, Danielsen B, Smith LH. Malignant melanoma in pregnancy. A population-based evaluation. Cancer. 2005;103(6):1217–26. https://doi.org/10.1002/cncr.20925.
107. Johansson AL, Andersson TM, Plym A, Ullenhag GJ, Moller H, Lambe M. Mortality in women with pregnancy-associated malignant melanoma. J Am Acad Dermatol. 2014;71(6):1093–101. https://doi.org/10.1016/j.jaad.2014.09.018.
108. Jones MS, Lee J, Stern SL, Faries MB. Is pregnancy-associated melanoma associated with adverse outcomes? J Am Coll Surg. 2017;225(1):149–58. https://doi.org/10.1016/j.jamcollsurg.2017.02.011.
109. Moller H, Purushotham A, Linklater KM, Garmo H, Holmberg L, Lambe M, Yallop D, Devereux S. Recent childbirth is an adverse prognostic factor in breast cancer and melanoma, but not in Hodgkin lymphoma. Eur J Cancer. 2013;49(17):3686–93. https://doi.org/10.1016/j.ejca.2013.06.047.
110. Byrom L, Olsen C, Knight L, Khosrotehrani K, Green AC. Increased mortality for pregnancy-associated melanoma: systematic review and meta-analysis. J Eur Acad Dermatol Venereol. 2015;29(8):1457–66. https://doi.org/10.1111/jdv.12972.
111. Kyrgidis A, Argenziano G, Moscarella E, Longo C, Alfano R, Lallas A. Increased mortality for pregnancy-associated melanoma: different outcomes pooled together, selection and publication biases. J Eur Acad Dermatol Venereol. 2016;30(9):1618. https://doi.org/10.1111/jdv.13202.
112. Martires KJ, Stein JA, Grant-Kels JM, Driscoll MS. Meta-analysis concerning mortality for pregnancy-associated melanoma. J Eur Acad Dermatol Venereol. 2016;30(10):e107–8. https://doi.org/10.1111/jdv.13349.

113. Tellez A, Rueda S, Conic RZ, Powers K, Galdyn I, Mesinkovska NA, Gastman B. Risk factors and outcomes of cutaneous melanoma in women less than 50 years of age. J Am Acad Dermatol. 2016;74(4):731–8. https://doi.org/10.1016/j.jaad.2015.11.014.
114. Martires KJ, Pomeranz MK, Stein JA, Grant-Kels JM, Driscoll MS. Pregnancy-associated melanoma (PAMM): Is there truly a worse prognosis? Would not sound alarm bells just yet. J Am Acad Dermatol. 2016;75(2):e77. https://doi.org/10.1016/j.jaad.2016.03.055.
115. de Haan J, Lok CA, de Groot CJ, Crijns MB, Van Calsteren K, Dahl Steffensen K, Halaska MJ, Altintas S, Boere IA, Fruscio R, Kolawa W, Witteveen PO, Amant F, International Network on Cancer I, Pregnancy. Melanoma during pregnancy: a report of 60 pregnancies complicated by melanoma. Melanoma Res. 2017;27(3):218–23. https://doi.org/10.1097/CMR.0000000000000327.
116. Reed KB, Brewer JD, Lohse CM, Bringe KE, Pruitt CN, Gibson LE. Increasing incidence of melanoma among young adults: an epidemiological study in Olmsted County, Minnesota. Mayo Clin Proc. 2012;87(4):328–34. https://doi.org/10.1016/j.mayocp.2012.01.010.
117. Keegan THM, Swetter SM, Tao L, Sunwoo JB, Clarke CA. Tumor ulceration does not fully explain sex disparities in melanoma survival among adolescents and Young adults. J Invest Dermatol. 2015;135(12):3195–7. https://doi.org/10.1038/jid.2015.325.
118. Daryanani D, Plukker JT, De Hullu JA, Kuiper H, Nap RE, Hoekstra HJ. Pregnancy and early-stage melanoma. Cancer. 2003;97(9):2248–53. https://doi.org/10.1002/cncr.11321.
119. MacKie RM, Bufalino R, Morabito A, Sutherland C, Cascinelli N. Lack of effect of pregnancy on outcome of melanoma. For the World Health Organisation melanoma Programme. Lancet. 1991;337(8742):653–5. https://doi.org/10.1016/0140-6736(91)92462-b.
120. McManamny DS, Moss AL, Pocock PV, Briggs JC. Melanoma and pregnancy: a long-term follow-up. Br J Obstet Gynaecol. 1989;96(12):1419–23. https://doi.org/10.1111/j.1471-0528.1989.tb06306.x.
121. Reintgen DS, McCarty KS Jr, Vollmer R, Cox E, Seigler HF. Malignant melanoma and pregnancy. Cancer. 1985;55(6):1340–4. https://doi.org/10.1002/1097-0142(19850315)55:6<1340::aid-cncr2820550630>3.0.co;2-t.
122. Slingluff CL Jr, Reintgen DS, Vollmer RT, Seigler HF. Malignant melanoma arising during pregnancy. A study of 100 patients. Ann Surg. 1990;211(5):552–7.; discussion 558-559. https://doi.org/10.1097/00000658-199005000-00005.
123. Wong JH, Sterns EE, Kopald KH, Nizze JA, Morton DL. Prognostic significance of pregnancy in stage I melanoma. Arch Surg. 1989;124(10):1227–30.; discussion 1230-1221. https://doi.org/10.1001/archsurg.1989.01410100133023.
124. Merkel EA, Martini MC, Amin SM, Yelamos O, Lee CY, Sholl LM, Rademaker AW, Guitart J, Gerami P. A comparative study of proliferative activity and tumor stage of pregnancy-associated melanoma (PAM) and non-PAM in gestational age women. J Am Acad Dermatol. 2016;74(1):88–93. https://doi.org/10.1016/j.jaad.2015.09.028.
125. Fabian M, Toth V, Somlai B, Harsing J, Kuroli E, Rencz F, Kuzmanovszki D, Szakonyi J, Toth B, Karpati S. Retrospective analysis of Clinicopathological characteristics of pregnancy associated melanoma. Pathol Oncol Res. 2015;21(4):1265–71. https://doi.org/10.1007/s12253-015-9961-4.
126. Beral V, Ramcharan S, Faris R. Malignant melanoma and oral contraceptive use among women in California. Br J Cancer. 1977;36(6):804–9. https://doi.org/10.1038/bjc.1977.265.
127. Gefeller O, Hassan K, Wille L. Cutaneous malignant melanoma in women and the role of oral contraceptives. Br J Dermatol. 1998;138(1):122–4. https://doi.org/10.1046/j.1365-2133.1998.02037.x.
128. Karagas MR, Stukel TA, Dykes J, Miglionico J, Greene MA, Carey M, Armstrong B, Elwood JM, Gallagher RP, Green A, Holly EA, Kirkpatrick CS, Mack T, Osterlind A, Rosso S, Swerdlow AJ. A pooled analysis of 10 case-control studies of melanoma and oral contraceptive use. Br J Cancer. 2002;86(7):1085–92. https://doi.org/10.1038/sj.bjc.6600196.
129. Tang JY, Spaunhurst KM, Chlebowski RT, Wactawski-Wende J, Keiser E, Thomas F, Anderson ML, Zeitouni NC, Larson JC, Stefanick ML. Menopausal hormone therapy and risks of melanoma and nonmelanoma skin cancers: women's health initiative randomized trials. J Natl Cancer Inst. 2011;103(19):1469–75. https://doi.org/10.1093/jnci/djr333.

130. Berk-Krauss J, Bieber AK, Criscito MC, Grant-Kels JM, Driscoll MS, Keltz M, Pomeranz MK, Martires KJ, Liebman TN, Stein JA. Melanoma risk after in vitro fertilization: a review of the literature. J Am Acad Dermatol. 2018;79(6):1133–40. e1133. https://doi.org/10.1016/j.jaad.2018.07.022.
131. Calderon-Margalit R, Friedlander Y, Yanetz R, Kleinhaus K, Perrin MC, Manor O, Harlap S, Paltiel O. Cancer risk after exposure to treatments for ovulation induction. Am J Epidemiol. 2009;169(3):365–75. https://doi.org/10.1093/aje/kwn318.
132. Hannibal CG, Jensen A, Sharif H, Kjaer SK. Malignant melanoma risk after exposure to fertility drugs: results from a large Danish cohort study. Cancer Causes Control. 2008;19(7):759–65. https://doi.org/10.1007/s10552-008-9138-5.
133. Stewart LM, Holman CD, Finn JC, Preen DB, Hart R. Association between in-vitro fertilization, birth and melanoma. Melanoma Res. 2013;23(6):489–95. https://doi.org/10.1097/CMR.0000000000000019.
134. Swetter SM, Tsao H, Bichakjian CK, Curiel-Lewandrowski C, Elder DE, Gershenwald JE, Guild V, Grant-Kels JM, Halpern AC, Johnson TM, Sober AJ, Thompson JA, Wisco OJ, Wyatt S, Hu S, Lamina T. Guidelines of care for the management of primary cutaneous melanoma. J Am Acad Dermatol. 2019;80(1):208–50. https://doi.org/10.1016/j.jaad.2018.08.055.
135. Driscoll MS, Grant-Kels JM. Hormones, nevi, and melanoma: an approach to the patient. J Am Acad Dermatol. 2007;57(6):919–31.; quiz 932-916. https://doi.org/10.1016/j.jaad.2007.08.045.
136. Peccatori FA, Azim HA Jr, Orecchia R, Hoekstra HJ, Pavlidis N, Kesic V, Pentheroudakis G, Group EGW. Cancer, pregnancy and fertility: ESMO clinical practice guidelines for diagnosis, treatment and follow-up. Ann Oncol. 2013;24(Suppl 6):vi160–70. https://doi.org/10.1093/annonc/mdt199.
137. Andtbacka RH, Donaldson MR, Bowles TL, Bowen GM, Grossmann K, Khong H, Grossman D, Anker C, Florell SR, Bowen A, Duffy KL, Leachman SA, Noyes RD. Sentinel lymph node biopsy for melanoma in pregnant women. Ann Surg Oncol. 2013;20(2):689–96. https://doi.org/10.1245/s10434-012-2633-7.
138. Gentilini O, Cremonesi M, Trifiro G, Ferrari M, Baio SM, Caracciolo M, Rossi A, Smeets A, Galimberti V, Luini A, Tosi G, Paganelli G. Safety of sentinel node biopsy in pregnant patients with breast cancer. Ann Oncol. 2004;15(9):1348–51. https://doi.org/10.1093/annonc/mdh355.
139. Nijman TA, Schutter EM, Amant F. Sentinel node procedure in vulvar carcinoma during pregnancy: A case report. Gynecol Oncol Case Rep. 2012;2(2):63–4. https://doi.org/10.1016/j.gynor.2012.01.003.
140. Ishida I, Yamaguchi Y, Tanemura A, Hosokawa K, Itami S, Morita A, Katayama I. Stage III melanoma treated with chemotherapy after surgery during the second trimester of pregnancy. Arch Dermatol. 2009;145(3):346–8. https://doi.org/10.1001/archdermatol.2008.612.
141. Amant F, Vandenbroucke T, Verheecke M, Fumagalli M, Halaska MJ, Boere I, Han S, Gziri MM, Peccatori F, Rob L, Lok C, Witteveen P, Voigt J-U, Naulaers G, Vallaeys L, Van den Heuvel F, Lagae L, Mertens L, Claes L, Van Calsteren K. Pediatric outcome after maternal Cancer diagnosed during pregnancy. N Engl J Med. 2015;373(19):1824–34. https://doi.org/10.1056/NEJMoa1508913.
142. Cardonick EH, Gringlas MB, Hunter K, Greenspan J. Development of children born to mothers with cancer during pregnancy: comparing in utero chemotherapy-exposed children with nonexposed controls. Am J Obstet Gynecol. 2015;212(5):658.e651. https://doi.org/10.1016/j.ajog.2014.11.032.
143. Grunewald S, Jank A. New systemic agents in dermatology with respect to fertility, pregnancy, and lactation. J Dtsch Dermatol Ges. 2015;13(4):277–89.; quiz 290. https://doi.org/10.1111/ddg.12596.
144. Mehta A, Kim KB, Minor DR. Case report of a pregnancy during Ipilimumab therapy. J Glob Oncol. 2018;4:1–3. https://doi.org/10.1200/JGO.17.00019.

145. Menzer C, Beedgen B, Rom J, Duffert CM, Volckmar A-L, Sedlaczek O, Richtig E, Enk A, Jäger D, Hassel JC. Immunotherapy with ipilimumab plus nivolumab in a stage IV melanoma patient during pregnancy. Eur J Cancer. 2018;104:239–42. https://doi.org/10.1016/j.ejca.2018.09.008.
146. Maleka A, Enblad G, Sjors G, Lindqvist A, Ullenhag GJ. Treatment of metastatic malignant melanoma with vemurafenib during pregnancy. J Clin Oncol. 2013;31(11):e192–3. https://doi.org/10.1200/JCO.2012.45.2870.
147. Pagan M, Jinks H, Sewell M. Treatment of metastatic malignant melanoma during pregnancy with a BRAF kinase inhibitor: a case report. Case Reports in Women's Health. 2019;24:e00142. https://doi.org/10.1016/j.crwh.2019.e00142.
148. de Haan J, van Thienen JV, Casaer M, Hannivoort RA, Van Calsteren K, van Tuyl M, van Gerwen MM, Debeer A, Amant F, Painter RC. Severe adverse reaction to Vemurafenib in a pregnant woman with metastatic melanoma. Case Reports in Oncology. 2018;11(1):119–24. https://doi.org/10.1159/000487128.
149. Altman JF, Lowe L, Redman B, Esper P, Schwartz JL, Johnson TM, Haefner HK. Placental metastasis of maternal melanoma. J Am Acad Dermatol. 2003;49(6):1150–4. https://doi.org/10.1016/S0190-9622(03)00124-5.
150. Schwartz JL, Mozurkewich EL, Johnson TM. Current management of patients with melanoma who are pregnant, want to get pregnant, or do not want to get pregnant. Cancer. 2003;97(9):2130–3. https://doi.org/10.1002/cncr.11342.
151. Alexander A, Samlowski WE, Grossman D, Bruggers CS, Harris RM, Zone JJ, Noyes RD, Bowen GM, Leachman SA. Metastatic melanoma in pregnancy: risk of transplacental metastases in the infant. J Clin Oncol. 2003;21(11):2179–86. https://doi.org/10.1200/jco.2003.12.149.

Chapter 8
Dermatologic Surgery in Pregnancy

Jennifer Villasenor-Park

Introduction

Dermatologic procedures during pregnancy can be safely performed with careful planning and consideration of risks to the patient and the fetus or infant. Factors such as timing of the procedure and possible risk with delay of treatment to the mother are all important considerations.

Timing

Timing of the procedure can significantly alter the risk to the fetus. The second trimester (weeks 13–24) is generally regarded as a relatively safe time to undergo a minimally invasive procedure [1, 2]. The first trimester, during which key organogenesis and possible spontaneous abortion are more likely to occur, and third trimester, during which preterm labor can occur, carry much higher risk for complications compared to the second trimester. However, it is important to weigh the relative risk for these complications and the risk for under treatment or delay in treatment of the patient.

J. Villasenor-Park (✉)
Department of Dermatology, University of Pennsylvania, Philadelphia, PA, USA

K. H. Tyler (ed.), *Cutaneous Disorders of Pregnancy*,
https://doi.org/10.1007/978-3-030-49285-4_8

Preoperative Considerations

Thorough preoperative assessment of the patient is essential and should include assessment of pregnancy-specific questions including a history of recent contractions, vaginal bleeding, abdominal pain, and edema. Additionally, assessment for possible preeclampsia is important. Any signs or symptoms of preeclampsia would be a contraindication and should prompt the surgeon to consult with the patient's obstetrician.

Intraoperative Considerations

Intraoperative considerations include optimal positioning for the safety of the patient and the fetus. Starting around week 20 during pregnancy, there is a greater risk for the gravid uterus to compress the inferior vena cava (IVC) leading to decreased venous return and cardiac output if patients are placed in the traditional supine position, which is known as aortocaval compression syndrome [3]. In patients not properly positioned, lightheadedness, nausea, vomiting, diaphoresis, hypotension, and tachycardia may occur as presenting signs of aortocaval compression syndrome. By placing the patient in the left lateral tilt position (Fig. 8.1) of 30°, compression of the IVC can be avoided [4, 5]. Examination of the gravid uterus and IVC by magnetic resonance imaging (MRI) have shown that the left lateral tilt position of 30° decreases compression of the IVC [6].

Antiseptics

In general, antiseptics considered safe for use during pregnancy include alcohol and chlorhexidine. Alcohol is commonly used for short procedures, such as skin biopsies. While it is percutaneously absorbed, it is rapidly metabolized and does not

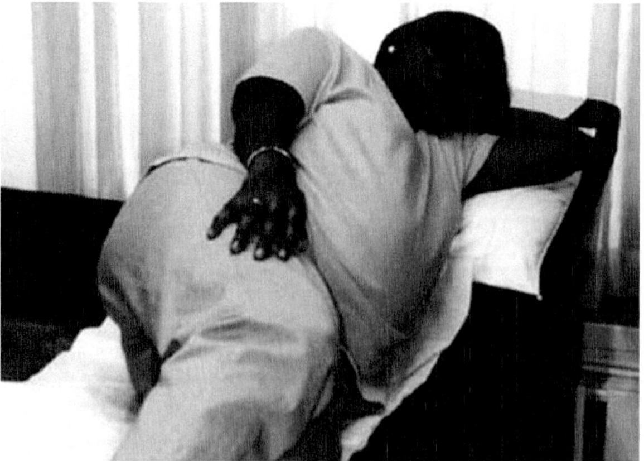

Fig. 8.1 Left lateral tilt position to prevent aortocaval compression syndrome in a pregnant patient

accumulate to significant levels in the blood [7]. For longer procedures, including excisions, chlorhexidine can be safely used during pregnancy [8]. Care should be taken to avoid sensitive areas such as the eye and ears due to the risk of corneal injury and ototoxicity [9, 10]. Povidine-iodine is avoided due to reports of neonatal hypothyroidism. Hexachlorophene is also avoided due to its association with severe fetal abnormalities [11].

Anesthesia

The anesthetic choice for pregnant patients should also be carefully considered. Lidocaine, which is widely used in dermatologic procedures, is considered safe for use during pregnancy in small amounts. There is no evidence to support harm to the fetus with the use of infiltrated lidocaine in animal studies; however, it does cross the placenta [12, 13]. The maximum safe dose of local infiltrative anesthesia with lidocaine is not known, but is suggested by the manufacturer to be 7 mg/kg of lidocaine with epinephrine and 4.5 mg/kg of lidocaine without epinephrine [13]. Doses of 3.0–4.5 mg/kg of lidocaine with epinephrine and 1.5–2.0 mg/kg of lidocaine without epinephrine appear to be safe in children [14, 15]. Although most dermatologic procedures rarely exceed these doses, lidocaine toxicity can occur if a large amount is inadvertently delivered intravascularly or if an idiosyncratic response occurs. Thus, careful monitoring for signs of lidocaine toxicity is important. Initial signs of lidocaine toxicity include perioral numbness, facial tingling, slurred or pressured speech, metallic taste, auditory changes and hallucinations, which may also accompany hypertension, tachycardia, and premature ventricular contractions. Cardiac and central nervous system toxicity progresses with increasing dose and can evolve to seizures, central nervous system depression, and can ultimately lead to cardiac failure or arrest [16]. Intravenous lipid infusion is used to prevent mortality secondary to lidocaine toxicity [17]. Bupivacaine and mepivacaine are generally not used in pregnant patients, as their use has been associated with inhibition of cardiac conduction, congenital abnormalities, and fetal bradycardia [1, 18]. Rare cases of methemoglobinemia from high dose prilocaine have been reported [5, 19].

Given its safe use as infiltrative local anesthesia, lidocaine is considered safe during pregnancy in the topical form as well [13]. Use of topical benzocaine is avoided due to the risk of methemoglobinemia in infants and children [20]. Lidocaine 2.5%/prilocaine 2.5% topical cream is considered safe for use during pregnancy but should not be used for long periods of time over large areas of the body due to the risk of methemoglobinemia with high doses of prilocaine [5, 19].

Epinephrine has been shown in one study to be associated with an increased risk of malformations in children of mothers exposed to systemic epinephrine during the first trimester [12]. Epinephrine can also decrease blood flow within the uterus, can potentially trigger uterine spasms, and reduce uterine contractile strength [21]. However, the concentration of epinephrine given via local infiltrative anesthesia is far below the concentration of epinephrine produced endogenously during stress and is unlikely to cause clinically significant adverse effects. Additionally, the local vasoconstrictive effects of epinephrine minimizes maternal blood concentration and placental transfer of lidocaine, thereby decreasing possible systemic toxicity from lidocaine to the mother and her baby [12]. The most recent guidelines for use of local anesthesia published by the American Academy of Dermatology indicate that small amounts of epinephrine in local infiltrative anesthesia may be safe for use during pregnancy [13].

Procedures during Pregnancy

Several studies have documented minimal significant change in the size, color and dermatoscopic features of nevi in pregnant women [22–28]. Dermatologists should use standard clinical and dermatoscopic guidelines when assessing melanocytic nevi in pregnant women. Therefore, any suspicious features noted in melanocytic nevi should not be attributed to a normal consequence of pregnancy. Skin biopsy can be safely conducted during any trimester of pregnancy and should not be delayed if there are suspicious melanocytic lesions noted during pregnancy. Use of lidocaine for local infiltrative anesthesia is considered safe for use during pregnancy [1]. While epinephrine has been associated with uterine artery spasm in animal and *in vitro studies*, the concentrations of epinephrine used during dermatologic surgery are considered safe and can reduce systemic absorption of lidocaine [1]. Diagnostic excisional biopsy by elliptical (fusiform) excision, punch excision, or deep shave/saucerization with narrow peripheral margins of 1–3 mm margins around the suspicious lesion is recommended [29].

Wide local excision with local anesthesia using appropriate margins for the treatment of melanoma can be safely conducted during pregnancy and should not be delayed once a diagnosis of cutaneous melanoma has been made [1, 29]. For patients with advanced stage melanoma, incorporation of a multidisciplinary group consisting of an obstetrician, dermatologist, surgeon and/or medical oncologist is important to provide optimal and appropriate care to pregnant women and is recommended in the most recent guidelines of care for the management of primary cutaneous melanoma published by the American Academy of Dermatology [29].

Sentinel lymph node biopsy is considered a safe, low-morbidity procedure that provides staging and prognostic information for patients with melanomas with a Breslow thickness of 1.0 mm or more and for thinner melanomas with high-risk features [30]. Timing of sentinel lymph node biopsy should be carefully considered to minimize risks to the mother and the fetus. In general, the sentinel lymph node biopsy may be safely performed during the second and third trimester. Isosulfan blue or lymphazurin is avoided due to the risk of severe allergic reaction and anaphylaxis [31–34]. Methylene blue is also avoided, particularly during the first trimester, due its known association with fetal abnormalities including atresia of the ileum and jejunum [35]. Use of technetium-99m (^{99m}Tc)-labeled radiocolloids in sentinel lymph node biopsy is considered safe during pregnancy because of its short half-life, and radioactive exposure delivered to the fetus is <0.01 Gy, which is well below the National Council on Radiation Protection and Measurement limits for a pregnant woman and the threshold dose of 0.1–0.2 Gy that is associated with increased risk of fetal malformation [1, 36]. In addition, the standard dose can be lowered without sacrificing radiographic information [37]. Sentinel lymph node biopsy should be avoided during the first trimester due to the risks associated with general anesthesia [29].

Treatment of non-melanoma skin cancer, such as basal cell carcinoma and squamous cell carcinoma, should be considered on an individual case-by-case basis, and the potential risks associated with treatment or delay of treatment should be discussed.

Elective procedures, including cosmetic procedures such as chemical peels and laser surgery, should be postponed to the postpartum period due to a lack of data regarding safety during pregnancy unless a compelling medical reason for treatment exists [5, 38]. Most data are limited to case reports of women treated during a time when they were not aware they were pregnant [5]. There are, however, several studies reporting the safe use of CO_2 laser therapy in the treatment of genital condyloma during pregnancy [39–42]. However, one report described the onset of premature rupture of membranes and subsequent delivery in one patient shortly after laser therapy and treatment with 85% trichloroacetic acid [43]. Use of other lasers during pregnancy have also been reported, but none have been studied for their safe use during pregnancy, so these procedures should be postponed until after pregnancy.

Postoperative Considerations

Acetaminophen is generally safe for use in the postoperative period for pregnant patients [1]. However, a case of acetaminophen poisoning resulting in fulminant hepatotoxicity and fetal demise was reported in a pregnant patient taking 9 grams per day for several days [44]. Patients should be advised to avoid exceeding the maximum recommended daily dose of 3 grams. Nonsteroidal anti-inflammatory drugs (NSAIDs) and salicylates are avoided during pregnancy due to their association with fetal cryptorchidism, low birth weight, and asthma [45, 46]. Further, the Federal Drug Administration (FDA) has advised women to discontinue use of NSAIDs and aspirin in the last 3 months of pregnancy due to the risk of renal injury, oligohydramnios, and premature close of the ductus arteriosus [1, 45].

Postoperative Infections

Treatment of postoperative infections should not be delayed in pregnant patients due to potential risks to the mother and fetus. Cephalosporins and penicillin are the most commonly prescribed medications for the treatment of cutaneous infections during the postoperative period and are both safe to use during pregnancy [47–49]. In patients who are unable to tolerate penicillin or cephalosporins, use of erythromycin, clindamycin, sulfonamides, and glycopeptides (vancomycin) may be considered [2, 48, 50]. While erythromycin is considered safe for use during the pregnancy, hepatoxicity can result from prolonged exposure to the estolate form [51]. There are also two studies that report an increase in atrial ventricular septal defects and pyloric stenosis if erythromycin is used during the first trimester [2, 48]. The data regarding safe use of sulfonamides and nitrofurantoin is somewhat mixed due to the potential risk of folate antagonism during the first trimester and subsequent development of birth defects when used with trimethoprim. However, according to the American College of Obstetricians and Gynecologists, their use is considered safe during all trimesters of pregnancy, particularly if there are no other safe alternative therapies [2, 48, 50]. Amongst aminoglycosides, streptomycin can lead to irreversible bilateral congenital deafness [2, 48, 52]. Fluoroquinolones should be avoided during pregnancy due to the risk of damage to bone and cartilage, renal toxicity, and cardiac defects [2, 48, 52, 53]. Following the 15th week of pregnancy, tetracycline use is not advised since it crosses the placenta, binds calcium, and causes enamel hypoplasia, discoloration of teeth, and inhibition of bone growth [48, 54].

Conclusions

Dermatologic procedures can be safely performed during pregnancy if all aspects of the procedure and the risks to the mother and fetus are carefully considered. While the 2nd trimester of pregnancy and postpartum period are the safest times to perform dermatologic procedures and are associated with the lowest risks to the fetus, the risk to the mother should treatment be delayed is also an important consideration. With thoughtful planning and consideration of all aspects of the procedure including pre- and post-operative care, medically necessary dermatologic procedures can be safely performed during all trimesters of pregnancy.

References

1. Li JN, Nijhawan RI, Srivastava D. Cutaneous surgery in patients who are pregnant or breastfeeding. Dermatol Clin. 2019;37(3):307–17. https://doi.org/10.1016/j.det.2019.03.002.
2. Tyler KH, Zirwas MJ. Pregnancy and dermatologic therapy. J Am Acad Dermatol. 2013;68(4):663–71. https://doi.org/10.1016/j.jaad.2012.09.034.
3. Jeejeebhoy FM, Morrison LJ. Maternal cardiac arrest: a practical and comprehensive review. Emerg Med Int. 2013;2013:274814. https://doi.org/10.1155/2013/274814.
4. Goldberg D, Maloney M. Dermatologic surgery and cosmetic procedures during pregnancy and the post-partum period. Dermatol Ther. 2013;26(4):321–30. https://doi.org/10.1111/dth.12072.
5. Lee KC, Korgavkar K, Dufresne RG Jr, Higgins HW 2nd. Safety of cosmetic dermatologic procedures during pregnancy. Dermatol Surg. 2013;39(11):1573–86. https://doi.org/10.1111/dsu.12322.

6. Higuchi H, Takagi S, Zhang K, Furui I, Ozaki M. Effect of lateral tilt angle on the volume of the abdominal aorta and inferior vena cava in pregnant and nonpregnant women determined by magnetic resonance imaging. Anesthesiology. 2015;122(2):286–93. https://doi.org/10.1097/ALN.0000000000000553.
7. Lachenmeier DW. Safety evaluation of topical applications of ethanol on the skin and inside the oral cavity. J Occup Med Toxicol. 2008;3:26. https://doi.org/10.1186/1745-6673-3-26.
8. Arifeen SE, Mullany LC, Shah R, Mannan I, Rahman SM, Talukder MR, Begum N, Al-Kabir A, Darmstadt GL, Santosham M, Black RE, Baqui AH. The effect of cord cleansing with chlorhexidine on neonatal mortality in rural Bangladesh: a community-based, cluster-randomised trial. Lancet. 2012;379(9820):1022–8. https://doi.org/10.1016/S0140-6736(11)61848-5.
9. Bever GJ, Brodie FL, Hwang DG. Corneal injury from presurgical chlorhexidine skin preparation. World Neurosurg. 2016;96:e610–4. https://doi.org/10.1016/j.wneu.2016.09.035.
10. Steinsapir KD, Woodward JA. Chlorhexidine keratitis: safety of chlorhexidine as a facial antiseptic. Dermatol Surg. 2017;43(1):1–6. https://doi.org/10.1097/DSS.0000000000000822.
11. Hailing H. Suspected link between exposure to hexachlorophene and malformed infants. Ann N Y Acad Sci. 1979;320(1):426–35. https://doi.org/10.1111/j.1749-6632.1979.tb56624.x.
12. Murase JE, Heller MM, Butler DC. Safety of dermatologic medications in pregnancy and lactation: part I. Pregnancy. J Am Acad Dermatol. 2014;70(3):e401–14; quiz 415. https://doi.org/10.1016/j.jaad.2013.09.010.
13. Kouba DJ, LoPiccolo MC, Alam M, Bordeaux JS, Cohen B, Hanke CW, Jellinek N, Maibach HI, Tanner JW, Vashi N, Gross KG, Adamson T, Begolka WS, Moyano JV. Guidelines for the use of local anesthesia in office-based dermatologic surgery. J Am Acad Dermatol. 2016;74(6):1201–19. https://doi.org/10.1016/j.jaad.2016.01.022.
14. Hancox JG, Venkat AP, Coldiron B, Feldman SR, Williford PM. The safety of office-based surgery: review of recent literature from several disciplines. Arch Dermatol. 2004;140(11):1379–82. https://doi.org/10.1001/archderm.140.11.1379.
15. Hancox JG, Venkat AP, Hill A, Graham GF, Williford PM, Coldiron B, Feldman SR, Balkrishnan R. Why are there differences in the perceived safety of office-based surgery? Dermatol Surg. 2004;30(11):1377–9. https://doi.org/10.1111/j.1524-4725.2004.30432.x.
16. Anesthesiologists SCoJSo (2019) Practical guide for the management of systemic toxicity caused by local anesthetics. Journal of Anesthesia 33(1):1–8. https://doi.org/10.1007/s00540-018-2542-4.
17. Neal JM, Woodward CM, Harrison TK. The American society of regional anesthesia and pain medicine checklist for managing local anesthetic systemic toxicity: 2017 version. Reg Anesth Pain Med. 2018;43(2):150–3. https://doi.org/10.1097/aap.0000000000000726.
18. Lee JM, Shin TJ. Use of local anesthetics for dental treatment during pregnancy; safety for parturient. J Dent Anesth Pain Med. 2017;17(2):81–90. https://doi.org/10.17245/jdapm.2017.17.2.81.
19. Hahn IH, Hoffman RS, Nelson LS. EMLA-induced methemoglobinemia and systemic topical anesthetic toxicity. J Emerg Med. 2004;26(1):85–8. https://doi.org/10.1016/j.jemermed.2003.03.003.
20. Friedman PM, Mafong EA, Friedman ES, Geronemus RG. Topical anesthetics update: EMLA and beyond. Dermatol Surg. 2001;27(12):1019–26. https://doi.org/10.1046/j.1524-4725.2001.01855.x.
21. Hood DD, Dewan DM, James FM 3rd. Maternal and fetal effects of epinephrine in gravid ewes. Anesthesiology. 1986;64(5):610–3. https://doi.org/10.1097/00000542-198605000-00011.
22. Akturk AS, Bilen N, Bayramgurler D, Demirsoy EO, Erdogan S, Kiran R (2007) Dermoscopy is a suitable method for the observation of the pregnancy-related changes in melanocytic nevi. J Eur Acad Dermatol Venereol 21(8):1086–90. https://doi.org/10.1111/j.1468-3083.2007.02204.x.
23. Gunduz K, Koltan S, Sahin MT, E EF (2003) Analysis of melanocytic naevi by dermoscopy during pregnancy. J Eur Acad Dermatol Venereol 17(3):349–51. https://doi.org/10.1046/j.1468-3083.2003.00792_2.x.
24. Nachbar F, Stolz W, Merkle T, Cognetta AB, Vogt T, Landthaler M, Bilek P, Braun-Falco O, Plewig G (1994) The ABCD rule of dermatoscopy. High prospective value in the diag-

nosis of doubtful melanocytic skin lesions. J Am Acad Dermatol 30(4):551–59. https://doi.org/10.1016/s0190-9622(94)70061-3.
25. Pennoyer JW, Grin CM, Driscoll MS, Dry SM, Walsh SJ, Gelineau JP, Grant-Kels JM (1997) Changes in size of melanocytic nevi during pregnancy. J Am Acad Dermatol 36(3 Pt 1):378–82. https://doi.org/10.1016/s0190-9622(97)80212-5.
26. Strumia R (2002) Digital epiluminescence microscopy in nevi during pregnancy. Dermatology 205(2):186–87. https://doi.org/10.1159/000063901.
27. Wyon Y, Synnerstad I, Fredrikson M, Rosdahl I (2007) Spectrophotometric analysis of melanocytic naevi during pregnancy. Acta Derm Venereol 87(3):231–37. https://doi.org/10.2340/00015555-0227
28. Zampino MR, Corazza M, Costantino D, Mollica G, Virgili A (2006) Are melanocytic nevi influenced by pregnancy? A dermoscopic evaluation. Dermatol Surg 32(12):1497–504. https://doi.org/10.1111/j.1524-4725.2006.32362.x.
29. Swetter SM, Tsao H, Bichakjian CK, Curiel-Lewandrowski C, Elder DE, Gershenwald JE, Guild V, Grant-Kels JM, Halpern AC, Johnson TM, Sober AJ, Thompson JA, Wisco OJ, Wyatt S, Hu S, Lamina T (2019) Guidelines of care for the management of primary cutaneous melanoma. Journal of the American Academy of Dermatology 80 (1):208-50. https://doi.org/10.1016/j.jaad.2018.08.055.
30. Crompton JG, Gilbert E, Brady MS. Clinical implications of the eighth edition of the American Joint Committee on Cancer melanoma staging. J Surg Oncol. 2019;119(2):168–74. https://doi.org/10.1002/jso.25343.
31. Cordeiro CN, Gemignani ML. Breast cancer in pregnancy: avoiding fetal harm when maternal treatment is necessary. Breast J. 2017;23(2):200–5. https://doi.org/10.1111/tbj.12780.
32. Cimmino VM, Brown AC, Szocik JF, Pass HA, Moline S, De SK, Domino EF. Allergic reactions to isosulfan blue during sentinel node biopsy–a common event. Surgery. 2001;130(3):439–42. https://doi.org/10.1067/msy.2001.116407.
33. Raut CP, Hunt KK, Akins JS, Daley MD, Ross MI, Singletary SE, Marshall GD Jr, Meric-Bernstam F, Babiera G, Feig BW, Ames FC, Kuerer HM. Incidence of anaphylactoid reactions to isosulfan blue dye during breast carcinoma lymphatic mapping in patients treated with preoperative prophylaxis: results of a surgical prospective clinical practice protocol. Cancer. 2005;104(4):692–9. https://doi.org/10.1002/cncr.21226.
34. Cragan JD. Teratogen update: methylene blue. Teratology. 1999;60(1):42–8. https://doi.org/10.1002/(sici)1096-9926(199907)60:1<42::Aid-tera12>3.0.Co;2-z.
35. Toesca A, Gentilini O, Peccatori F, Azim HA Jr, Amant F. Locoregional treatment of breast cancer during pregnancy. Gynecol Surg. 2014;11(4):279–84. https://doi.org/10.1007/s10397-014-0860-6.
36. Pandit-Taskar N, Dauer LT, Montgomery L, St Germain J, Zanzonico PB, Divgi CR. Organ and fetal absorbed dose estimates from 99mTc-sulfur colloid lymphoscintigraphy and sentinel node localization in breast cancer patients. J Nucl Med. 2006;47(7):1202–8.
37. Adelstein SJ. Administered radionuclides in pregnancy. Teratology. 1999;59(4):236–9. https://doi.org/10.1002/(SICI)1096-9926(199904)59:4<236::AID-TERA9>3.0.CO;2-6.
38. Trivedi MK, Kroumpouzos G, Murase JE. A review of the safety of cosmetic procedures during pregnancy and lactation. Int J Women's Dermatol. 2017;3(1):6–10. https://doi.org/10.1016/j.ijwd.2017.01.005.
39. Arena S, Marconi M, Frega A, Villani C. Pregnancy and condyloma. Evaluation about therapeutic effectiveness of laser CO2 on 115 pregnant women. Minerva Ginecol. 2001;53(6):389–96.
40. Chaisilwattana P, Bhiraleus P. Carbon dioxide laser vaporization for genital wart. J Med Assoc Thail. 1996;79(12):749–54.
41. Gay C, Terzibachian JJ, Gabelle C, Reviron S, Ramanah R, Mougin C. Carbon dioxide laser vaporization of genital condyloma in pregnancy. Gynecol Obstet Fertil. 2003;31(3):214–9. https://doi.org/10.1016/s1297-9589(03)00040-7.
42. Wozniak J, Szczepanska M, Opala T, Pisarska-Krawczyk M, Wilczak M, Pisarski T. Use of CO2 laser in the treatment of condylomata acuminata of the anogenital region in pregnant women. Ginekol Pol. 1995;66(2):103–7.

43. Schwartz DB, Greenberg MD, Daoud Y, Reid R. Genital condylomas in pregnancy: use of trichloroacetic acid and laser therapy. Am J Obstet Gynecol. 1988;158(6 Pt 1):1407–16. https://doi.org/10.1016/0002-9378(88)90375-4.
44. Thornton SL, Minns AB. Unintentional chronic acetaminophen poisoning during pregnancy resulting in liver transplantation. J Med Toxicol. 2012;8(2):176–8. https://doi.org/10.1007/s13181-012-0218-2.
45. Bloor M, Paech M. Nonsteroidal anti-inflammatory drugs during pregnancy and the initiation of lactation. Anesth Analg. 2013;116(5):1063–75. https://doi.org/10.1213/ANE.0b013e31828a4b54.
46. Nezvalova-Henriksen K, Spigset O, Nordeng H. Effects of ibuprofen, diclofenac, naproxen, and piroxicam on the course of pregnancy and pregnancy outcome: a prospective cohort study. BJOG. 2013;120(8):948–59. https://doi.org/10.1111/1471-0528.12192.
47. Ailes EC, Gilboa SM, Gill SK, Broussard CS, Crider KS, Berry RJ, Carter TC, Hobbs CA, Interrante JD, Reefhuis J, National Birth Defects Prevention Study. Association between antibiotic use among pregnant women with urinary tract infections in the first trimester and birth defects, National Birth Defects Prevention Study 1997 to 2011. Birth Defects Res A Clin Mol Teratol. 2016;106(11):940–9. https://doi.org/10.1002/bdra.23570.
48. Tyler KH. Dermatologic therapy in pregnancy. Clin Obstet Gynecol. 2015;58(1):112–8. https://doi.org/10.1097/GRF.0000000000000089.
49. Watson M, Geller AC, Tucker MA, Guy GP, Weinstock MA (2016) Melanoma burden and recent trends among non-Hispanic whites aged 15–49years, United States. Preventive Medicine 91:294-298. https://doi.org/10.1016/j.ypmed.2016.08.032.
50. Committee opinion no. 717: sulfonamides, nitrofurantoin, and risk of birth defects. Obstet Gynecol. 2017;130(3):e150–2. https://doi.org/10.1097/aog.0000000000002300.
51. Kallen B, Danielsson BR. Fetal safety of erythromycin. An update of Swedish data. Eur J Clin Pharmacol. 2014;70(3):355–60. https://doi.org/10.1007/s00228-013-1624-3.
52. Bookstaver PB, Bland CM, Griffin B, Stover KR, Eiland LS, McLaughlin M. A review of antibiotic use in pregnancy. Pharmacotherapy. 2015;35(11):1052–62. https://doi.org/10.1002/phar.1649.
53. Kaguelidou F, Turner MA, Choonara I, Jacqz-Aigrain E. Ciprofloxacin use in neonates: a systematic review of the literature. Pediatr Infect Dis J. 2011;30(2):e29–37. https://doi.org/10.1097/INF.0b013e3181fe353d.
54. Leachman SA, Reed BR. The use of dermatologic drugs in pregnancy and lactation. Dermatol Clin. 2006;24(2):167–97, vi. https://doi.org/10.1016/j.det.2006.01.001.

Conclusion

In this age of targeted treatments and rapid development of novel immune-mediated therapies, it is challenging to stay up to date. There has never been a more critical time to ensure all healthcare professionals treating obstetric patients have a thorough knowledge of all currently available medication safety data.

Despite the challenges inherent in treating pregnant patients, becoming informed about skin disease and medication safety in pregnancy can assist physicians and healthcare providers with making appropriate treatment decisions for both the mother and fetus. The authors have provided a thorough review of normal physiologic skin changes in pregnancy, pregnancy-specific dermatoses, common pre-existing skin conditions not specific to pregnancy, skin cancer in pregnancy, proper use of dermatologic surgery during pregnancy, and specific information about treatment and medication safety for each condition. Please use this book as a valuable resource as you move forward with treating this unique patient population.

K. H. Tyler (ed.), *Cutaneous Disorders of Pregnancy*,
https://doi.org/10.1007/978-3-030-49285-4

Index

A

Acetaminophen, 117
Acne during pregnancy, 78, 79
  cosmetic treatment
    laser, 82
    phototherapy, 82
  diagnosis, 77
  epidemiology, 76
  pathophysiology, 76, 77
  systemic treatment options
    antibiotics, 81
    hormonal therapy, 82
    isotretinoin, 81, 82
    spironolactone, 81
    zinc, 82
  topical treatment options
    antibiotics, 80
    azelaic acid, 79
    benzoyl peroxide, 79
    glycolic acid, 80
    retinoids, 80, 81
    salicylic acid, 79
    sodium sulfacetamide, 80
  treatment, 77
Acne vulgaris, 76
Acute urticaria, 18
Acyclovir, 67
Adapalene, 80
Allergic and irritant contact dermatitis, 22
Androgenetic alopecia (AGA), 7
Anesthesia, 115, 116
Antenatal atopy, 62
Anti-androgen therapy, 82
Antibiotics, 81
Antihistamines, 23, 67, 68
Antiseptics, 114, 115
Anti-tumor necrosis factor (TNF) agents, 46
Aortocaval compression syndrome, 114
Atopic dermatitis (AD) of pregnancy
  clinical presentation, 60
  diagnosis, 60
  epidemiology, 59
  pathogenesis, 60, 61
  treatment, 62, 69–70
    acyclovir, 67
    antihistamines, 67, 68
    azathioprine, 66, 67
    cyclosporine, 65, 66
    dupilumab, 66
    methotrexate, 68
    mycophenolate, 68
    phototherapy, 63
    psoralens, 68
    systemic antibiotics, 67
    systemic corticosteroids, 64, 65
    topical antibiotics, 64
    topical calcineurin inhibitors, 64
    topical corticosteroids, 63
    unsafe agents, 68
Atopic eruption of pregnancy (AEP)
  clinical presentation, 20, 21
  definition, 19
  differential diagnosis, 22
  epidemiology, 19
  pathogenesis, 20
  pathology, 22
  treatment, 21–23
Attention deficit disorder, 62

K. H. Tyler (ed.), *Cutaneous Disorders of Pregnancy*,
https://doi.org/10.1007/978-3-030-49285-4

Autoimmune connective tissue diseases, 51
  cutaneous lupus erythematous, 51
    disease activity, 52
    pregnancy outcomes, 52, 53
    treatment, 53, 54
  dermatomyositis, 54, 55
    disease activity, 55
    pregnancy outcomes, 55
    treatment, 56
Autoimmune progesterone dermatitis, 22
Azathioprine, 66, 67
Azelaic acid, 6, 79, 84
Azithromycin, 67, 81

B
Basal cell carcinoma, 89, 90
Benzocaine, 115
Benzoyl peroxide (BPO), 79
BRAF inhibitors, 101
Broadband ultraviolet B phototherapy (BBUVB), 82
Bullous pemphigoid (BP), 28
Bupivacaine, 115

C
CO_2 laser therapy, 117
Catagen, 7
Cephalosporins, 67, 81, 117
Cetirizine, 68
Chemotherapy, 100, 101
Chloroquine, 54
Chlorpheniramine, 68
Chronic urticaria, 18
Clindamycin, 81, 117
Contact dermatitis, allergic and irritant, 22
Corticosteroids, 84
Cosmetic procedures, 117
Cutaneous changes during pregnancy, 75, 76
Cutaneous lupus erythematous, 51
  disease activity, 52
  pregnancy outcomes, 52, 53
  treatment, 53, 54
Cutaneous melanoma, 116
Cutaneous T-cell lymphoma (CTCL), 91
Cyclophosphamide, 54
Cyclosporine (CSA), 46, 65, 66

D
Demodex mites, 83
Dermatofibrosarcoma protuberans, 91
Dermatologic surgery
  anesthesia, 115, 116
  antiseptics, 114, 115
  intraoperative considerations, 114
  postoperative considerations, 117
  postoperative infections, 117, 118
  preoperative considerations, 113
  procedures during pregnancy, 116, 117
  timing, 113
Dermatomyositis (DM), 54, 55
  disease activity, 55
  pregnancy outcomes, 55
  treatment, 56
Diffuse red patches, 15
Diphenhydramine, 68
Direct immunofluorescence (DIF), 16
Discoid lupus erythematosus (DLE), 51
Discoid lupus of the chest, 52
Down syndrome, 82
Drug eruptions, 22
Dupilumab, 66
Dysplastic nevus syndrome, 92

E
Eccrine function, 11
Eczema herpeticum, 62
Elective procedures, 117
Epinephrine, 115, 116
Erythematotelangiectatic rosacea, 84
Erythromycin, 81, 84, 117
Erythromycin ethylsuccinate, 81
Estrogen, 24, 93
Estrogen receptor alpha (ERα), 93
Estrogen receptor beta (ERβ), 93
E-type atopic eruption of pregnancy, 20
E-type eczematous patches, 21
European Task Force on Atopic Dermatitis (ETFAD), 66
Evidence-based guidelines, 63
Extraocular sebaceous carcinoma, 90

F
Federal Drug Administraion (FDA), 78
Fetal deoxyribonucleic acid, 14
Fetal morbidity, 25
First-generation antihistamines, 68
5α-dihydrotestosterone (5α-DHT), 77
Fluoroquinolones, 118
Fluticasone propionate, 63

G
Glycolic acid, 80
Glycopeptides, 117
Gottron's papules, 55

Granuloma gravidarum, 9, 10
Gravid uterus, 10

H
Hemorrhoid(s), 10
Hemorrhoidal varicosities, 10
High factor broad spectrum sunscreens, 5
Hirsutism, 8
Hormonal therapy, 82
Hormone replacement therapy (HRT), 99
Human chorionic gonadotropin (hCG), 76, 90
Human Leukocyte Antigen (HLA), 94
Hydroxychloroquine (HCQ), 53, 56
Hyperandrogenism, 77
Hyperpigmentation, 3

I
Immunogloblulin E (IgE), 60
Immunoglobulin G1 (IgG1) antibody, 100
Immunoglobulin G4 (IgG4) antibody, 100
Impetigo herpetiformis (IH), 44
Inferior vena cava (IVC), 114
Inflammatory cascade of rosacea, 83
International Network on Cancer, Infertility, and Pregnancy (INCIP), 97
Intradermal eosinophils, 15
Intrahepatic cholestasis of pregnancy
  clinical presentation, 25
  definition, 23
  differential diagnosis, 26
  epidemiology, 24
  pathogenesis, 24, 25
  pathology, 26
  treatment, 26, 27
Intrauterine growth restriction (IUGR), 53
Intravenous lipid infusion, 115
In-utero corticosteroid, 65
Ipilimumab, 100
I-Pledge program, 82
Isotretinoin, 81, 82

K
Kaposi sarcoma, 90, 92
Keratinocyte carcinomas, 89

L
Lasers, 82
Lidocaine, 115
Linea alba, 3
Linea nigra, 3, 4
Loratadine, 68
Lupus erythematosus, 51–54

M
Macrolides, 81
Major Histocompatibility Complex (MHC)II molecules, 27
Maternal atopic dermatitis, 62
Mechanical tension, 6
Melasma, 4–6
Mepivacaine, 115
Merkel cell carcinoma (MCC), 90
Merkel cell polyomavirus (MCV), 90
Methemoglobinemia, 115
Methotrexate, 48, 68
Molluscum fibrosum gravidarum, 7
Montgomery tubercles, 11
Mupirocin, 64
Mycophenolate, 68
Mycophenolate mofetil (MMF), 54, 68
Mycosis fungoides (MF), 91

N
Nail growth, 8
Narrative FDA System, safety of drugs during pregnancy and lactation, 78
Narrowband ultraviolet B phototherapy (NBUVB), 23, 46, 82
Neonatal intensive care unit (NICU), 101
Nivolumab, 100
Non-melanoma skin cancer, 89–92, 117
Nonsteroidal anti-inflammatory drugs (NSAIDs), 117

O
Ocular rosacea, 84
Oral contraceptive pills (OCPs), 99

P
Palmar erythema, 9
Papulopustular rosacea, 84
Pembrolizumab, 100
Pemphigoid gestationis (PG), 14
  clinical presentation, 28, 29
  definition, 27
  differential diagnosis, 30
  epidemiology, 27
  pathogenesis, 27, 28
  pathology, 29, 30
  treatment, 30
Penicillin, 67, 81, 117

Periumbical plaques, 29
Perivascular inflammatory infiltration, 17
Photoprotection, 56
Phototherapy, 63, 82
Phymatous rosacea, 84
Pigmentary demarcation lines, 4
Polycystic ovarian syndrome (PCOS), 77
Polymorphic eruption of pregnancy (PEP)
  clinical presentation, 15, 16
  definition, 13
  differential diagnosis, 17, 18
  epidemiology, 14
  pathogenesis, 14, 15
  pathology, 16
  treatment, 17–19
Postpartum hair shedding, 7
Povidine-iodine, 115
Prednisolone, 64
Prednisone, 64
Pregnancy
  physiologic skin changes in, 3
    connective tissue changes, 6, 7
    glandular activity, 11
    hair and nail changes, 7, 8
    pigmentary changes, 3–6
    vascular changes, 9, 10
  pre-existing skin disease in, 43–49
Pregnancy dermatoses
  atopic eruption of pregnancy
    clinical presentation, 20, 21
    definition, 19
    differential diagnosis, 22
    epidemiology, 19
    pathogenesis, 20
    pathology, 22
    treatment, 21–23
  intrahepatic cholestasis of pregnancy
    clinical presentation, 25
    definition, 23
    differential diagnosis, 26
    epidemiology, 24
    pathogenesis, 24, 25
    pathology, 26
    treatment, 26, 27
  pemphigoid gestationis
    clinical presentation, 28, 29
    definition, 27
    differential diagnosis, 30
    epidemiology, 27
    pathogenesis, 27, 28
    pathology, 29, 30
    treatment, 30
  polymorphic eruption of pregnancy
    clinical presentation, 15, 16
    definition, 13
    differential diagnosis, 17, 18
    epidemiology, 14
    pathogenesis, 14, 15
    pathology, 16
    treatment, 17–19
Prilocaine, 115
Probiotics, 67
Propionibacterium acnes (*P. acnes*), 76, 80
Pruritic folliculitis of pregnancy (PFP), 20
Pruritus, 26
Psoralen plus ultraviolet A light phototherapy (PUVA), 48
Psoralens, 68
Psoriasis, 43
  biologic therapy, considerations for, 47
  biologics, 47
  disease activity of, 43, 44
  pregnancy outcomes in, 44
  steroids, 45
  therapeutics, 48
  treatment, 45–47
P-type atopic eruption of pregnancy, 20
Pustular psoriasis of pregnancy (PPP), 44
Pyoderma faciale, 83
Pyogenic granuloma, 9

R
Regulatory T cells (Tregs), 94
Retinoids, 5
Rosacea during pregnancy
  diagnosis, 84
  epidemiology, 83
  pathophysiology, 83
  subtypes, 84
  treatment, 84
Rosacea fulminans (RF), 83, 84

S
Salicylates, 117
Salicylic acid, 79
Sebaceous gland activity, 11
Sebum, 77
Second-generation antihistamines, 68
Sentinel lymph node biopsy, 116
Sex hormone binding globulin (SHBG), 77
Sex steroid, 4
Skin cancer in pregnancy
  melanoma, 93, 94
    diagnosed before or after pregnancy, 98, 99
    diagnosis, 94–98

exogenous hormones, 99
family planning, 101, 102
nevi, pregnancy associated changes in, 92, 93
treatment, 100, 101
non-melanoma skin cancer, 89–92
Sodium sulfacetamide, 80
Spider angiomata, 9
Spironolactone, 81
Squamous cell carcinoma, 89
Staphylococcus aureus infections, 62
Streptomycin, 118
Striae gravidarum, 6, 7
Subcutaneous lupus erythematosus (SCLE), 51
Sulfonamides, 117
Superficial micronodules of pregnancy, 92
Suprabasal keratinocytes, 14
Systemic antibiotics, 67, 77
Systemic azithromycin, 84
Systemic corticosteroids, 64, 65

T
Telangiectasias, 82
Telogen effluvium, 7, 8
Tetracyclines, 81
Toll-like receptor (TLR), 83
Toll-like receptor 2 (TLR2) signaling, 83
Topical antibiotics, 64, 77, 80
Topical calcineurin inhibitors, 64
Topical corticosteroids, 63
Topical dapsone, 80
Topical metronidazole, 84
Topical mupirocin, 64
Topical retinoids, 80, 81
Topical steroid, 63
Topical tazarotene, 80
Toxic epidermal necrolysis (TEN), 101
Tretinoin, 5, 6, 80
Tumor necrosis factor (TNF) α, 83
Type 1 T helper cells (Th1), 76

U
Ursodeoxycholic acid, 26
Urticarial plaques, 15, 29
US Food and Drug Administration (FDA) Drug Risk Classification System for Pregnant Women, 78
Ultraviolet A phototherapy, 68

V
Vancomycin, 117
Vascular endothelial growth factor (VEGF), 83
Vemurafenib, 101
Venous hypertension, 10
Venous varicosities, 10
Viral hepatitis, 26
Voigt/Futcher lines, 4

X
Xerosis cutis, 22

Z
Zinc, 82

GPSR Compliance

The European Union's (EU) General Product Safety Regulation (GPSR) is a set of rules that requires consumer products to be safe and our obligations to ensure this.

If you have any concerns about our products, you can contact us on ProductSafety@springernature.com

In case Publisher is established outside the EU, the EU authorized representative is:

Springer Nature Customer Service Center GmbH
Europaplatz 3
69115 Heidelberg, Germany

Batch number: 10372213

Printed by Printforce, the Netherlands